STOP
BACK PAIN!

STOP BACK PAIN!

Prevent, reduce and eliminate
back pain for good!

Simon Fox

Library of Congress Control Number:		2017916693
ISBN:	Hardcover	978-1-5434-0466-1
	Softcover	978-1-5434-0465-4
	eBook	978-1-5434-0464-7

To order additional copies of this book, contact:
Xlibris
1-800-455-039
www.Xlibris.com.au
Orders@Xlibris.com.au
749410

CONTENTS

Stop Back Pain

Prevent, reduce, and eliminate back pain for good

Simon Fox, BSc (Hons), Dip. Remedial Massage, Dip. Fitness, Exercise Coach, and Exercise Rehabilitation Specialist

Self-belief is something I struggled with as I have worked to complete this book. But it's true that I have the education, experience, and knowledge on this topic to help and inspire you to live your life without back pain. Thank you to all those people who have believed in me and supported me along the way.

FOREWORD

BACK PAIN IS one of the most debilitating injuries or conditions a person can have. Statistics show that over 85 per cent of the population will suffer from a bout of back pain at some stage in their lives. Unfortunately, a large percentage of these people never fully recover, living the rest of their lives in constant aches and pain. Please understand this is *not* normal, and you shouldn't accept it.

The majority of people who suffer from back pain are usually on a roller-coaster ride, having a low-grade pain or stiffness daily with a debilitating episode occurring once or twice a year. This usually depends on activity levels and workload. There's no reason for anyone to suffer from back pain. Whether you have a disc bulge, a prolapse, or a major injury, this pain can be reduced and even eliminated.

The aim of this book is to teach you how to live your life pain-free. Our goal is to educate you on why roller-coaster rides happen and how to get off. If you can live pain-free for one minute, then you should be able to go pain-free for an hour or even a year.

Reading this book won't cure your back pain. In fact, *just reading* this book won't do anything to reduce your pain. *You need to take action.*

The first section of this book will help you understand why a lot of treatments don't give you long-term relief. Then we will look at different types of back pain and why people suffer from them. Finally, we'll teach you basic techniques and strategies we have developed and used to help eliminate back pain.

Action is the key. One of the worse things you can do is *not move.* The other worst thing you can do is the *wrong type of movement.* Let us educate you so you're armed with easy-to-understand theories and facts on how to best strengthen your back.

It's less common in today's medical world for people with back pain to be advised to stop moving. However, if you have back pain and you have been given this advice, please find a new medical professional to advise you. The body is designed to move; the worst thing you can do for lower back pain is to stop moving.

This book is about empowering you with knowledge and exercises so you can develop a strong, healthy back. I have written this book using real-life case studies of people whom I have seen in my private practice. I'll use these scenarios to explain the anatomical and physiological concepts behind their back pain. Furthermore, I'll discuss the treatment plan and exercises used to treat them.

Of course, we need to have a waiver. Please note that everyone is different, and although a case study may sound like your situation, it doesn't mean that the treatment applied to them will work for you. Please feel free to apply any or all the theories presented. However, we do strongly recommend that you seek guidance from a health professional.

Live life with quality, not pain. If you would like advice, have questions related to the theory concepts in this book, or wish to arrange a consultation either via Skype or in person, please contact our administration at info@lifestyleessentials.com.au.

Knowledge is power. To control your body, you need knowledge.

Click here to see our welcome video to our book, we hope this book helps you eliminate back from your life
http://stopbackpain.com.au/introduction-to-back-pain-book

TURN OFF YOUR PAIN

BEFORE GETTING INTO the first chapter, it is essential to give you something to help reduce your pain. If you're suffering back pain right now, let's help you straight away rather than waiting until the end of the book.

The first step in starting any type of back pain program is to turn off the pain and return the body to a relaxed state. This can be done through the nervous system. I'll explain this in further detail later in the book. Below are two simple exercises that will help you turn off your pain. Do these exercises two or three times a day, and you'll see a reduction in your pain levels within a few days.

Tip No. 1: (Transverse Abdominis) TVA Breathing

Breathing is one of the simplest activities we do in life. Yet so many people breathe incorrectly. The correct technique is termed 'diaphragmatic breathing'. As you breathe in, your stomach should push out first, and then your chest should expand. A lot of people only breathe from their chest. You can see this in more detail on our *Back Pain Eliminator* DVD series.

Click or scan the link below to watch a video on
how to do your TVA breathing exercise
https://www.stopbackpain.com.au/stop-back-pain-correct-breathing

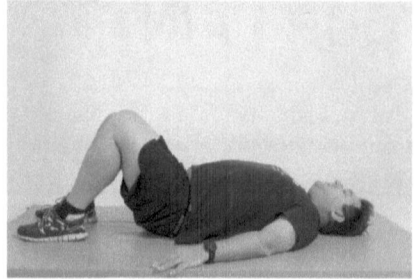 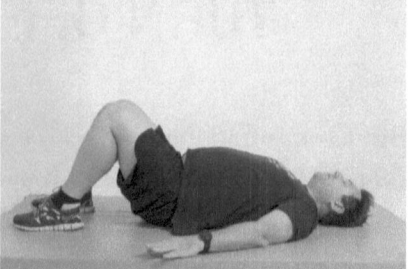

Breathe in (bloated stomach)   *Breathe out (stomach draws in)*

More of these videos and exercises can be obtained through
www.stopbackpain.com.au/stop-back-pain-exercise-videos

Tip No. 2: TVA Four-Point Stance (Decompression)

This is my 'go to' exercise to help people reduce back pain. Just placing yourself in this position will help reduce your pain. More importantly, ensure that you're in a quiet environment; don't have the kids jumping on you. You need to focus on your breathing while doing this exercise. Kneel on the floor on all fours, and try to develop what is termed a 'neutral spine'.

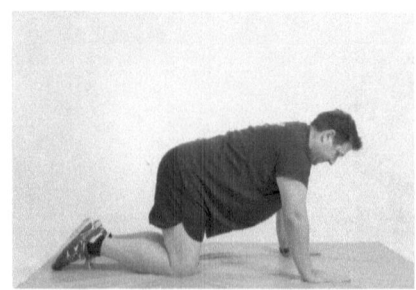 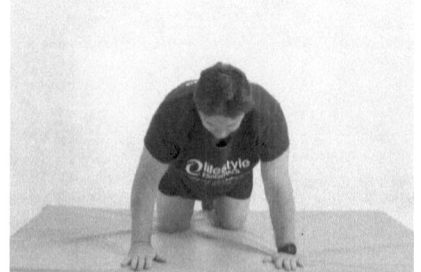

Attempt to develop a neutral spine. (You might need a mirror.) Become familiar with the position of the body so that you can repeat it.

Activate your TVA by drawing in your abdominals.

Take the weight out of the opposite arm and leg, but keep the hand and knee in contact with the floor.

Alternate from one side to the other, taking the weight out of the opposite arm and leg.

Try not to let the hips rotate or move. Keep them straight and still.

A TICKING BOMB

UNFORTUNATELY, MOST SERIOUS back injuries occur later in the evening, when you're picking up a tissue or something light or just going to the bathroom. This is when you're more dehydrated, fatigued, and just not thinking about protecting your back; in other words, it's when you least expect it.

Is your back a ticking bomb? Do you live life in fear of your back giving out? Not participating in activities in case you'll hurt your back?

> Mrs Jones was 39 years of age; by all accounts a fit and healthy female with no children. She had a fall and hurt her back. After treating her over a period of time, we have successfully reduced the pain, but unfortunately she has regular twinges and back aches. The memory of the pain, and the fear of having her back pain return, impacted her on a number of levels. Firstly, she adapted her lifestyle so she wouldn't do anything 'to upset her back'. She was living in constant fear of her back pain returning and this prevented her from participating in many activities, even when her back didn't hurt.

This constant fear of reinjuring your back leads to two problems. One, you let the fear of back pain control you. Two, you tend to move as though you're in pain to protect yourself. Both of these are reasonable responses.

Once the body is in pain, it tends to respond to that injury in a particular way. This response will usually be a movement or posture that causes the least amount of pain. This action is driven by the pain, placing the body into positions that are the most comfortable. Unfortunately, when a person continues to put their body into this pain-driven posture, the body may turn on the pain mechanism again.

Think of your posture as a switch. Pain switches on a postural response, and your posture can (and will) switch on your pain pathways.

You need to turn off the time bomb. The first step is to make the decision not to be in pain. Even when you're in pain, make that decision not to be in pain. You do this by consciously taking proactive steps to reduce and eliminate the pain. Secondly, don't let your pain define you. Yes, you suffer from back pain, but you're not defined by it. Don't let it control you. A good example is the person who states, 'I'm a diabetic' or 'I have back pain/sciatica.' By making this statement, you're claiming the condition defines you. If you're defined by this, you won't be able to get rid of it because it's part of your identity, and no one wants to lose their identity. Changing your language and making your pain or health problem a 'thing' rather than a part of you is a big step to psychologically not hold on to the pain. We discuss this concept more in the next chapter.

I don't believe in back pain. Yes, this is a big statement. I'm not saying it doesn't exist, nor am I saying that I don't occasionally have a sore back. But by making this statement, it means that psychologically I don't accept back pain. When I have a sore back, that's all it is – a sore back. I know what to do to eliminate the pain, and I just do it. This is often enough to make the pain disappear. Remember that you reap what you sow, and what you focus on is what you'll often achieve. By stating that you suffer from back pain or that you're in constant pain, then the chances are high that you'll be in constant pain, even though you don't want it.

THE MIND GAME

YOUR MIND IS the most powerful tool you have in determining your health and pain levels. Just make the decision to be pain-free, and let the mind do its job. Remember, 'ask and you shall receive.'

Back pain is real. At no stage do I ever deny that back pain isn't real or doesn't exist. Pain is real too. At no stage in twenty years of clinical practice have I ever said or agreed with any type of pain being in the mind. This chapter is about understanding that pain is something you *have* and not letting it define who you are. It's essential to never let your back become your identity.

There are a number of social media groups about back pain. People can join these groups to discuss their condition and look for new ideas they can use to help overcome their pain. However, what occurs in a large percentage of these groups is that they become a place where people simply discuss their back pain story, reliving the injury, the surgery, and the pain over and over again like a badge of honour. They compete with one another to see who has the worse condition, but there's a serious problem in living this way.

Tony Robbins, inspiration speaker and motivator, talks about the effect a person's physiology has on their psychology, thus affecting how they feel, act, and react. When you relive your back pain *story* with other people, this can psychologically and emotionally cause you to relive *your pain*, setting off the psychological and, in turn, neurological processes that cause pain.

When the body becomes injured or is in pain, it reacts in a number of ways. There's a musculoskeletal response, an immune system response to aid in healing, a neurological response which normally drives the pain, and a psychological response. The last response is a protective one, where the body forms a memory of the injury and the pain in an attempt to prevent it from occurring again. When a person continues to verbally and emotionally share their back pain story with other people, they can often trigger the psychological memory of the injury which then triggers the physiological pain. Your pain pathways fire up, leading to a relapse or an increase in your pain levels.

One of the major causes of long-term back pain is when you allow your condition to define you. Your identity is an extremely powerful part of who you are. When you let a disease or a condition such as back pain shape part of your identity, it's extremely hard to eliminate that pain. This is because if you lose the back pain, you also lose part of your identity.

If you suffer from back pain and continue to talk about and relive your condition, injury, or surgical procedure(s) with other people, there's a strong possibility that your condition will become part of your identity. If you wish to be pain-free, you need to break this psychological connection now. Let's set up a three-stage process to break this:

1. Stop all talk and thought process about having back pain or a back condition. A simple way is changing your words from 'I have back pain' to 'I do suffer from back pain on occasions.' This can be taken a step further by stating, 'I sometimes suffer from a sore back.' By changing the words, you're able to change the strength of the psychological connection. Therefore it doesn't become embedded into your neural pathways as being part of you.

2. Set up a positive statement that declares you're not in pain. This is Psychology 101. It's called a self-fulfilling prophecy, meaning that what you believe about yourself will shape your behaviour. This behaviour will then drive the outcome to match the belief. In relation to back pain, I draw on an example of a person's posture. If you suffer from back pain (and maybe you do) but you also *believe* it, then you'll move in a way and take on a postural position that will support that belief, and your back pain continues. By changing your belief to 'I don't suffer from back pain', you prevent the body's neurological processes from going into postural positions that cause pain.

3. When a professional is treating you and helping you overcome long-term chronic pain such as that associated with back pain, it's all about your belief system. If you don't believe it will work, then it won't – simple. You need to believe in your treatment plan; this psychological process of believing will prevent the negative old neurological pain pathways from being psychologically triggered.

Self-belief is the biggest aspect to everything in life. *If you believe you can, you're right. If you believe you can't, you're right.*

What do you believe when it comes to your back? The reality is that your mind is one of the most powerful tools a therapist has to work with in helping you overcome your pain. So let's use it the right way.

LONG-TERM RELIEF

WHEN YOU SUFFER from back pain, you seek treatment, but who should you see? Most GPs will refer you to a physiotherapist, but there are so many other alternatives now available in the medical world. These include chiropractic, osteopathy, myotherapy, remedial massage, Bowen therapy, Chinese medicine, and exercise physiology. Because of this long list, you would think it would be easy to find a program that eliminates your pain. Unfortunately, this is not often the case; clients coming into our clinic have suffered from back pain for years and never received any long-term relief.

There are people who swear by their practitioner, seeing them every two to four weeks to maintain their backs so they can be pain-free. This is great, especially if they're truly pain-free. But I would argue that all they're doing is maintaining their back and preventing painful symptoms rather than treating the cause of the pain. Do you want to maintain your back or live pain-free?

Today's society seems to have been sold on the idea that living in pain is normal and that degeneration of our health is just part of the aging process. This is totally untrue. Refuse to accept it, and if you're ever told this by any health professional or specialist, find a new one. It's only in extreme circumstances that you might expect to live with long-term pain and may need to manage this pain because your condition can't be treated. This type of situation (where pain management techniques are necessary) is normally related to conditions that require surgical intervention. It's my opinion, based on clinical experience, that every back injury or condition treated with the right rehabilitation program will see a significant reduction in pain.

Seeing a therapist is a key part of any back pain elimination program. The reality is that if you have back pain or symptoms related to it, you require treatment. This will help the muscles, tendons, ligaments, nerves, and connective tissues to function correctly and help your body take on a better biomechanical position, enabling you to at least attempt to function normally. When you start with a therapist, they will see you at least once or twice a week. But they should have a treatment plan, which they'll discuss with you. The duration between visits increases as your pain becomes reduced.

If these two things aren't happening and your therapist can't explain why, then you need to find a new one. A treatment plan should reduce the symptoms and pain and address the cause of the problems.

Get off the treatment merry-go-round. Needing to see a therapist every 2–6 weeks is *not* a remedy; it's a Band-Aid.

If you have found a practitioner who works well with you, that's great news; stick with them. But what does 'working well with you' actually mean? You ultimately go to an allied health professional for help with a significant long-term reduction of pain, which is partnered with an increase in mobility and functionality. Remember that there are *good* and *great* therapists. Accept that a great therapist will ask you questions and answer your questions; if you can't get the answers, seek a second opinion.

In every rehabilitation program, there will be relapses and incidences where the pain returns. However, each time this happens, you should see a reduction in the severity of pain and experience a quicker recovery.

What Is the why?

Symptoms aren't the cause. The types of pain you may experience include sciatic pain, a dull to more intense ache and/or pain in your back, and headache, which are termed 'symptoms'. These symptoms occur in response to a condition. For example, if you have a prolapsed disc, the vertebra will often rub, or even trap, a nerve coming out of your spine. Its location in the spine will determine where you experience the pain and other symptoms, such as numbness in one or both legs or groin pain.

Example 1

John came into the clinic with long-term back pain. He rated his pain as an 8 out 10. He has been seeing another therapist for a number of weeks and not had any improvement or relief. His symptoms included sciatic pain down his leg as well as a stabbing pain in the lower back. After an assessment, I determined that John had tight muscles in his lower back. However, he also had an uneven hip height as well as what presented as an uneven leg length. After the initial treatment, we found that a number of muscles in his pelvic region weren't working correctly, leading to the instability of his pelvis, causing hip and leg length instability.

Now from a treatment perspective, if I had only treated the sciatic symptoms by loosening up the muscles in the lower back, pelvis, and hamstrings, he would have had some relief. But it would have only been for a short while. The key to an effective treatment plan is for the therapist to be capable of explaining the 'why' behind the back pain; without the why, they're only treating the symptoms.

There are many, many reasons why a person can have lower back pain. The pain will present in specific ways, depending on the reason, so it's essential that the therapist assesses your whole body to learn why you have pain in your back.

Example 2

Annie has had lower back pain on and off for the last fifteen years. She had gotten to the stage where she believed she just had to live with the pain and manage it with painkillers. When we assessed her, we asked her about injuries she had had in the past in limited detail. One that she told us about was an old ankle injury. She said she had rolled her ankle twenty years ago and that it didn't cause her any pain or other problems. Further examination showed that her ankle was extremely limited in its movement, although not causing pain.

The problem with this is that the ankle does affect the hip, and if it's not working correctly, the hip will become dysfunctional too. This, in turn, causes back pain. So by treating the ankle, we fix the back.

You must have a therapist who looks at the whole body, not just the areas in pain. A full understanding comes from looking at the whole body, not just the bits that hurt.

A lot of back pain treatment plans don't work. This can often be because the therapist is treating the symptoms rather than the cause. It can also be because you need to take a holistic approach. It's extremely rare that one therapist can treat back pain and provide long-term relief. You need a team of medical people who specialise in their own areas to effectively overcome back pain.

Do you only hire a builder to build a house? No. You hire an electrician for wiring, a plumber for the water, a painter for the painting, and so on. Everyone has a specific role to play in building the house. This is the same method used when treating a person for back pain. To effectively stop the pain in the long term, you need a team of therapists who can work with you to move you forwards.

What do you need to effectively treat back pain? Firstly, you need a therapist who can treat you. They should be able to treat the soft tissue, as well as offer some joint mobilisation. It would also be ideal for them to understand the nervous system so they can help you turn off the pain and desensitise your nervous system. Secondly, you need someone who understands what correct posture is and what type of exercises you should do to correct any neural muscular imbalances. Finally, you need someone who can teach you how to strengthen the body in the correct way so you can continue to function at an optimal level.

TYPES OF BACK PAIN

THERE ARE MANY different reasons why people suffer from back pain. Though there may be hundreds of specific conditions leading to this type of pain, all of them will fall into two main categories, structural and functional problems.

Structural abnormalities are caused by abnormal features of the bone(s) or between the bones. An example is an abnormally shaped bone or joint or damage to a bone or disc such as a fracture or prolapse. These types of problems usually require surgery to relieve the pain, and the surgeon may be able to remove some of the abnormalities, although this isn't always successful. Having this type of problem does *not* condemn you to a life of pain. Implementing the correct rehabilitation program and ensuring that the body is correctly supported will reduce pain and dysfunction.

Functional abnormalities are imbalances, weaknesses, incorrectly loading, or postural problems that are caused by how we function in life. An example of this type of problem is when a person has an overcurvature in their spine from using a computer or when specific muscles are dysfunctional and tight. These types of problems are more common and can be treated by implementing the correct combination of therapy, mobilisation, strengthening, and stretching.

When seeing a medical professional, people tend to fall into one of two situations. The first situation is where the health professional has an explanation for the cause of your pain. You have a clear understanding of what you need to do to reduce and eliminate the pain. This problem will usually lead you to see an allied health professional such as a physiotherapist, an osteopath, or a chiropractor regularly to maintain your back and quality of life. Whether or not this works long term is another thing.

The second situation is where you've had numerous consultations, scans, and tests, yet there's nothing wrong with you. You're in constant pain that prevents you from being able to function. The worst thing about it is that everyone says there's nothing wrong, yet you're in pain. The reality is that there *is* something wrong; it's just that the medical world hasn't been able to establish what it is.

The majority of these cases are caused by postural imbalances, muscular weaknesses, or the body not functioning correctly, leading to incorrect loading of the back, hips, and pelvis. Living with this idiopathic back pain plays mind games with you. However, you need to accept that something *is* causing the problem, and you must keep seeking out therapists who can assess you and help you identify the cause of your pain.

Structural Causes of Back Pain

Rob came to the clinic looking to improve his ability to function. He knew his back pain could not be fixed as he had bone spurs growing into the spinal canal. When these irritate the spinal cord, he suffers sciatica and significant back pain. Training him was a challenge, knowing we couldn't fix his back. What we didn't expect was that by strengthening the lower back and abdominal muscles, as well as getting him moving, we saw a dramatic decrease in his pain to the extent that he put off surgery and now plays with the kids again.

Structural causes of back pain are just that – abnormalities or changes to the make-up of the body that can't be nonsurgically changed. For many years, it has been accepted that you can't help people with structural issues. Any sort of treatment is to keep them moving in an attempt to reduce the pain. Over the last 2–3 years, we have clinically learned that by mobilising and strengthening the body correctly, there will be a major decrease in structurally caused pain to the point where they can live their life pain-free.

In 2004, I trained a client who had structural scoliosis (lateral deviation of the spine, seen in figure 1) as a personal trainer. This condition occurred in her early adolescence. It was so bad that they surgically implanted steel rods down either side of her spine. If they didn't do this, she would have died. She suffered pain all the time. But by participating in a regular strength training program focused on strengthening her back muscles and

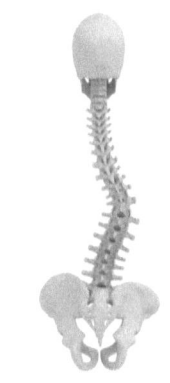

Figure 1. Lateral curvature of the spine.

abdominal muscles, she would often report that she had no pain. The right exercise program will reduce the pain and help you function pain-free daily.

Functional Causes of Pain

Functional back pain is a much larger area of discussion. It's where pain is caused by problems that have arisen through your body, and these can include

- postural imbalances,
- disc and joint problems,
- general wear and tear on the spine,
- muscle imbalances, and
- joint immobility.

Unfortunately, a lot of these functional problems (if not treated) can lead to structural damage. For example, poor posture that leads to incorrect loading of the spine can cause a bulged disc. If this isn't corrected, the bulge may weaken and become a prolapsed disc, which is now a structural problem.

Posture Counts

'Sit up straight,' 'Don't slouch,' and 'You need to improve your posture' are common statements made during your childhood and adolescence. What is correct posture? What is normal? To eliminate back pain and to improve your posture, you first need to understand what correct posture really is.

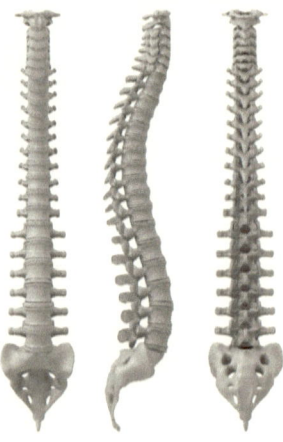

Figure 2. Vertebral column – five sections of the spine.

The spine is made up of *five major sections*. Each section has a specific function. The shape and structure of each of these regions of the spine determines its structure and function. For example, the lower back is the weight-bearing region, so it has larger vertebra bodies. The neck's function is related to mobility, so it has less bony processes, allowing a larger range of movement. Therefore the spine's ability to move or stabilise is dependent on its structure (figure 2).

WHAT IS A NEUTRAL SPINE?

THE SPINE IS not straight. It has five natural curves that allow it to function normally and weight-bear correctly in supporting the body. These natural curves are referred to as a 'neutral spine'.

The Cervical Region (Neck)

The top region is the neck, also known as the cervical spine. The major function of the neck is to support and allow a large range of movement of the head. The neck is the most mobile part of the spine. This region is essential for the normal functioning of the neck. As you can see in figure 3, the neck is not straight. It has what's termed a lordotic curve. This curve forms a convex shape and can straighten out when you spend too much time in front of a computer or when your head protrudes forwards. When this occurs, people will often suffer from headaches, migraines, and a lack of mobility in the neck. Dysfunction in the neck may lead to shoulder problems, including numbness and muscle weakness in the arms and shoulders.

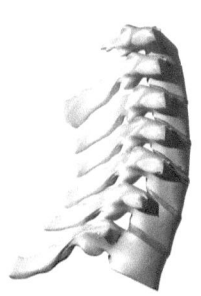

Figure 3. Cervical spine.

The posture of the neck and the position of the head will also affect other regions of the body. When the head is too far forwards, it will increase the load on the neck as seen below. This forces the muscles and connective tissues to work harder to support the head. This increase in load will often lead to further imbalances in other regions of the spine. In the diagram below, you can see that as the head moves further forwards, the curvature on the rest of the spine changes. This will lead to imbalances and possible weaknesses further down the spine.

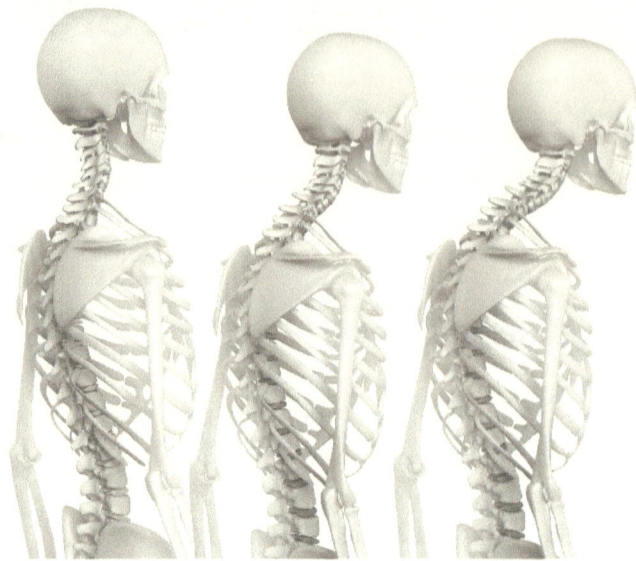

Figure 4. Different positions of head carriage.

The further the head protrudes forwards from the body, the greater the load will be that gets transferred into the neck and its muscles (figure 4).

Thoracic Region

The next region of the spine forms the ribcage and is termed the thoracic

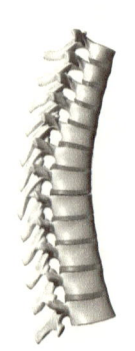

Figure 5. Thoracic vertebral spine.

spine. This area makes up the thoracic cage (the ribs), sternum, and vertebrae. The role of the thoracic cage is to protect the heart, lungs, liver, and kidneys. The major movements that occur are bending forwards and backwards, although this backward movement is limited. There is limited rotation in this area because of where the ribs attach to the vertebral bodies. The thoracic region has a natural concave-shaped curve. This curvature of the spine is termed a kyphotic curve. When this curve is excessive, it creates a hunchback-type posture.

Lumbar Region

The lower back is termed the lumbar spine. This is the main weight-bearing portion of the spine. The main movement in this area is rotational, although it will allow some forward and backward bending. From a back pain perspective, this is where the majority of dysfunction occurs. Injuries such as prolapsed discs and disc bulges are more common here than in other regions of the spine.

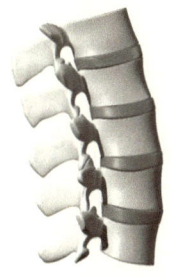

Figure 6. Lumbar vertebral spine.

Sacrum and Coccygeal Region

Sacrum and coccygeal bones form what is commonly known as the tail bone. These two regions are formed by fused bones, and it stops any movement between each individual bone. The sacrum and the iliac bone of the pelvis form a joint called the sacroiliac (SI) joint. This joint connects the vertebral column (base of the spine) to the pelvis. The primary function of the sacroiliac joint is for shock absorption. It's a moveable joint allowing only 2–4 mm of movement. As you age or if there's an increase in the wear and tear on the joint, its ability to move decreases as it becomes stiff and 'locked'. This type of dysfunction can lead to a number of problems with the pelvis, hips, legs, and spine. Some of these issues include muscle imbalance, nerve impingement, osteopubitis, leg length discrepancies, poor posture, and incorrect loading in the spine. Furthermore, it can lose its ability to provide shock absorption, increasing the load carried by the spine.

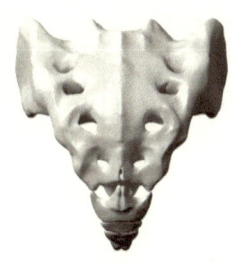

Figure 7. Sacral and coccygeal vertebra.

GOOD POSTURE CREATES GOOD HEALTH

YOUR SPINE (POSTURE) forms the foundation of your health. In fact, your posture is able to affect nearly every system in the body. The vertebral column is the housing for the spinal cord. At each level of the vertebral column is a pair of spinal nerves (see figure). These nerves innervate organs and systems in the body, such as the immune system, cardiac system, and respiratory system. In fact, the spinal nerves are the major connection points for the parasympathetic nervous system (PNS) and the sympathetic nervous system (SNS). These are the two main nervous systems that determine the body's response to its surrounding environment. These are the fight-or-flight systems. The figure below shows the impact that each of the nervous systems have on the body and its systems.

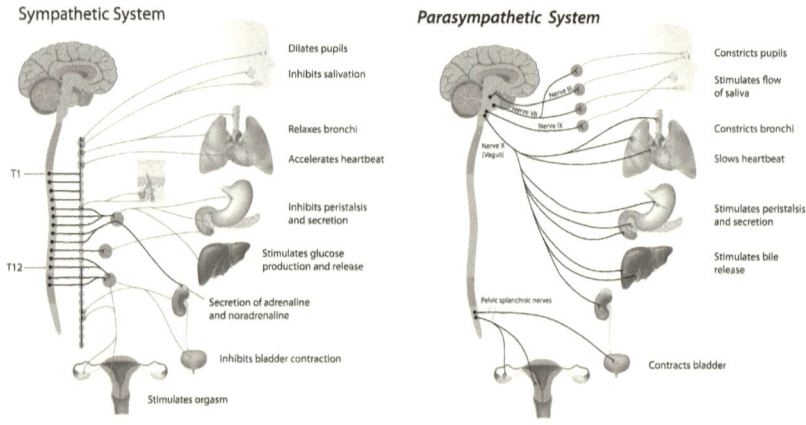

Figure 8. The parasympathetic and sympathetic nervous systems control the body's pain mechanisms.

Incorrect alignment of the spine through injury, dysfunction, or just poor posture can cause the nerves that leave the spine to become impinged. When this occurs, it can be like turning a light switch on or off. Think of the nervous system as the electrical wiring of the body. When a nerve becomes trapped or isn't able to function normally, it's either stimulated to function too much or inhibited so that it does not function at all. Either way, it can have a negative impact on the overall ability of the body to function.

An example of this type of neurological response occurred with a client in 2003. I have a male client named Bob, who came to the clinic. He had midback pain and neck tightness. At the time of the appointment, there were other medical issues. However, the night after the massage, the client was rushed to hospital thinking that he was having a heart attack, but he hadn't. Then a few weeks later, after his next massage, he ended up in the hospital again, suffering from a racing heartbeat and palpitations. After about three months of tests and visits back and forth to the hospital, it was discovered that he had a prolapsed disc in the seventh thoracic vertebra. The treatment loosened up the muscles around this area and caused an irritation of the nerve that affected his heart and heart rate, causing him to experience heart-attack-like symptoms post-treatment. Needless to say, the treatment plan had to change.

This example demonstrates how an injury in the spine can cause downstream effects on the body. In this example, the cardiovascular system was affected. There have been many other times when postural imbalances in the lower back have affected digestion, the reproductive system, and even the immune system.

The ideal curvature in your upper (thoracic) and lower (lumbar) back is between thirty and thirty-five degrees. If the curves aren't in this range, it doesn't necessarily mean you'll have problems, but it may increase the risk of developing problems in the future. When it comes to posture, the most important aspect is the ability of a person to function pain-free. If a person has what's termed a 'normal posture' yet it's functional, then you should run with it rather than try to make huge changes.

ABNORMAL CURVES
CAUSE BACK PAIN

ABNORMAL CURVES OF the spine cause incorrect loading of the spine, muscle tightness, neurological hypersensitivity, and pain. When looking at abnormal curvatures of the spine, there can be an overcurvature and/or a loss of curvature of the spine. Both issues can cause back pain.

Scoliosis is when there's a lateral deviation of the spine – the curve is sideways. The curvature forms an S shape left to right (or right to left) rather than front to back. Structural scoliosis is when there's an abnormality in the shape of the bones, or they grow the wrong way. This type of scoliosis may need to be assessed by a spinal specialist and may also require surgery, especially if it's a child still growing.

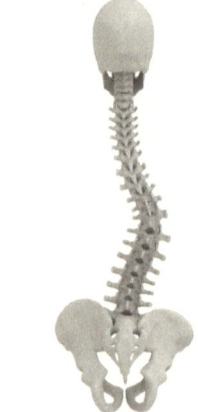

Figure 9. Scoliosis is a lateral curvature of the spine.

Functional scoliosis can be caused by a number of issues, including postural imbalances, tight muscles, uneven leg length, and instability of the SI joint. Regardless of the cause, it's always associated with muscle tightness, especially in the regions that are pulled together.

In figure 5, you can see the sideways shifting of the vertebral column. If this is due to muscle tightness (workstation not set up correctly or sitting on your wallet), then stretching or treating these muscles with manual therapy, such as massage or dry needling, should help relieve the muscles and allow the spine to readjust itself.

Another common cause of scoliosis is uneven leg length. This can occur in two ways. You may have an anatomical difference in the length of the leg bones, or the hip joint isn't sitting correctly, leading to a difference in leg length.

Scoliosis (which is caused by structural abnormalities) is often unable to be changed, and the best outcome for this person is to develop a good treatment strategy to keep the back muscles strong to help stabilise the spine, thus keeping the pain to a minimum.

Problems associated with scoliosis include the following:

- hip pain
- unstable pelvis
- ankle problems
- uneven leg length
- knee pain
- nerve impingement
- muscle imbalances
- muscular tightness
- pain

EXCESSIVE KYPHOSIS

KYPHOSIS IS THE normal curvature of the upper region of the back. Excessive kyphosis (or hunched back) is an overcurvature of this upper back region (the thoracic spine). This problem can lead to a number of complaints, including tightening of the chest muscles, numbness and pins and needles in hands, carpal-tunnel-like symptoms, forward head carriage, stiffness in the neck, loss of neck mobility, shoulders rolled forwards, and shoulder pain, with conditions such as bursitis and developing frozen shoulder.

Excessive kyphosis can often affect other curves in the spine. Forward head carriage tends to accompany excessive kyphosis. This is when the head protrudes forwards, over time causing ongoing neck problems. The secondary problem is it moves your centre of gravity forwards. This means the majority of the weight is now in front of the spine. Your spine will often compensate for this by increasing the curve of the lower back in an attempt to keep the body weight balanced.

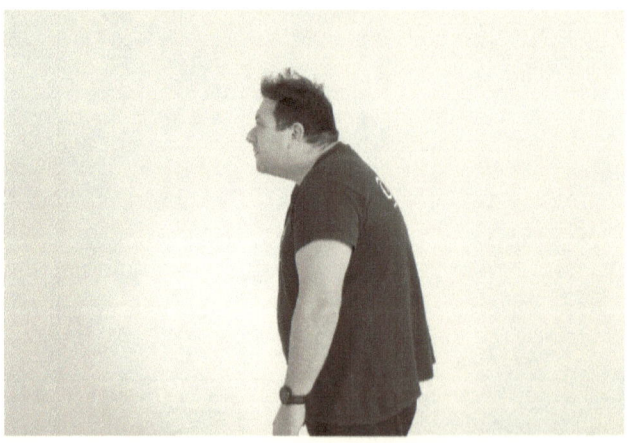

Figure 10. Excessive kyphosis is often partnered with forward head carriage and shoulders rolled forwards.

The diagram demonstrates an excessive kyphotic spine.

Problems associated with excessive kyphosis include the following:

- tightness of the chest
- reduced lung capacity (shortness of breath)
- rolling forwards of the shoulders
- numbness and pins and needles in the arm and hands
- thoracic outlet syndrome
- frozen shoulder
- bursitis of the shoulder
- muscle weakness in the upper back
- lower back pain
- neurological hypersensitivity
- forward head carriage
- headaches and migraines
- excessive curvature of the lower spine
- hamstring problems
- calf problems and Achilles tendon tightness

Unfortunately, the whole body isn't assessed most of the time. A therapist tends to focus on the symptoms such as Achilles tendon issues (being a calf problem) rather than look at the whole structure and ask, 'Why are these tight?'

EXCESSIVE LORDOSIS

LORDOSIS IS THE normal curve in the lower back as seen in the figure below. When this curve is too large, it's referred to as excessive lordosis. Excessive loading of the front of the body, as seen in pregnant women or people who are excessively overweight, often develops to counterbalance the excessive weight. When this curve becomes too large, it can lead to a number of secondary problems such as nerve impingement, tight muscles in the lower back, pelvis issues, knee pain, disc problems, excessive wear and tear on the spine, and sciatica. An excessive curve in this region can lead to other postural issues with the hip and pelvic areas.

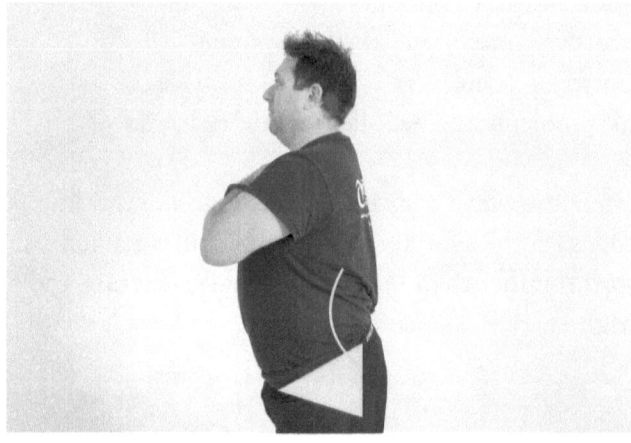

Figure 11. Excessive lordosis is often accompanied by an anterior pelvic tilt.

The picture demonstrates excessive lordosis of the lumbar spine.

Problems associated with excessive lordosis include the following:

- nerve impingement (leading to chronic pain)
- incorrect loading of the intervertebral discs
- disc bulges
- prolapsed discs
- sciatica

- hip dysfunction (tightness and pain)
- overcurvature of the thoracic region
- weak abdominals
- tight hamstrings and calves
- knee pain (patellar tracking issues)
- Achilles tendon problems
- ankle dysfunction

The spine forms the central foundation for the whole body; it's the concrete and the framework. Everything is affected by your spinal posture. As you can see, incorrect posture can lead to systematic dysfunction as well as secondary issues in other regions such as the pelvis and lower limbs. Unlike your mobile phone, your television, and even your heart, you can't just get a new spine when you damage or wear out the one you have. You need to look after it because it's the only one you have for the rest of your life. Yes, there are surgical interventions to help people with spinal problems, but none are that effective, so it's smarter to prevent the problem in the first place.

Are you ready to become proactive and improve the posture of your spine? If not, chances are high that by the time you're in your late fifties, you'll have a list of ailments causing you pain and dysfunction. The good news is most of these imbalances are reversible if treated correctly and early enough.

ELIMINATE BACK PAIN: TURN OFF THE PAIN

KNOW PAIN, KNOW *gain.* The first step in eliminating back pain is understanding it. Once you do understand it, you can reduce it and then, ultimately, turn it off. Long-term pain is when a person has constant pain for more than twelve weeks. Long-term or chronic pain is a much more complex level of pain to deal with because the nervous system is involved in controlling the pain, not just the injury.

Neurologically, the body will respond to your world in one of two ways; it prepares the body for action or for a resting, relaxed state. The nervous system that prepares you for action is termed the sympathetic nervous system, and it's designed to respond to and deal with stress. Its major role is to prepare the body for fight or flight. When this nervous system is switched on, there's an increase in your heart rate, your breathing will become faster and shallower, your vision is sharper, and you have better auditory acuity. Your body's senses are turned on, and more specifically, their sensitivity is turned up.

Pain is a sympathetic nervous system response. This nervous system is the one that drives pain by increasing the sensitivity of the pain receptors. It responds by increasing muscle tension around the injured area in an attempt to protect the body.

> **Your sympathetic nervous system**
> An example of this is the first time you are home alone at night as a child. You hear a noise, and your heart rate increases, and your hearing becomes more sensitive. You look outside to see what you have heard, and you see all the trees moving and the shadows in the dark.

The second nervous system is the parasympathetic one. It turns us off, allowing bodily functions such as digestion, growth, and repair. When this system is activated, your breathing slows, and muscle tension is more relaxed.

These two systems can't work at the same time. When one is on, the other is off. So if you're living a high-stress life, you're setting your nervous system up to support an injury state and, possibly, even long-term pain.

How to Turn off Your Sympathetic Nervous System

One of the best ways to turn off this nervous system is to turn on the parasympathetic nervous system. Meditation, breathing, and relaxation-based activities are effective. I suggest the half-foam roller breathing exercise. Lie on a foam roller so the roller is along your spine, making sure your head and spine is on the foam roller, and just lie. Focus on breathing in really slowly for 3–5 seconds and then out for 3–5 seconds. If your mind jumps, let it happen, but just keep focusing on your breathing. If you're a type A personality (like me), it will take a while before you're able to do it, but it *will* work. Once you're in this relaxed state, it will turn off your sympathetic nervous system, allowing your parasympathetic to switch on.

Credit to Mark Buckley for this exercise (www.fmastrengthtraining.com).

STAGES OF PAIN

WHEN YOU INJURE yourself, the body goes through a healing process. Muscles usually take 2–4 weeks to heal, while tendons and ligaments can take up to 12 weeks. These time frames will vary depending on the treatment plan. Ice prevents bleeding, while heat enhances blood flow, which leads to healing. In the recovery phase, the more heat you can keep on the injured area, the quicker it will heal.

There are two types of pain:

1. *Acute pain* is the pain that occurs from the healing process. Tissues are damaged. There are swelling, inflammation, and other cellular mechanisms involved in the healing process, which often cause pain.
2. *Chronic pain* is the type of pain that occurs when the healing process is finished and is usually due to neurological effects.

Negative Feedback Loop

What happens when a person has a long-term injury to their back? The first response of the nerves in the injured area is to communicate with the brain about the injury, saying 'ouch'. This message will be in the form of pain but may be numbness, stabbing pain, a dull ache, or burning sensation.

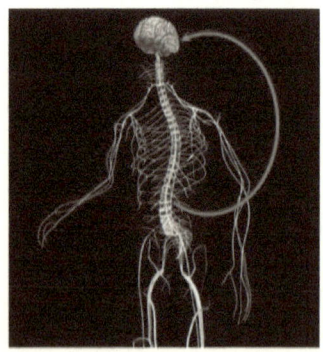

Figure 12. Pain in the lower back is communicating an 'ouch' message to the brain.

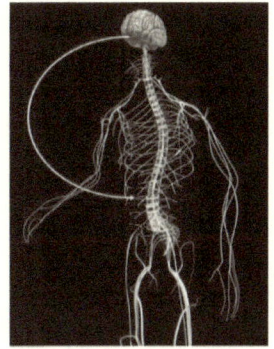

Figure 13. *Brain sends a message to the muscles in the lower back to not move.*

The brain then communicates with all the muscles, tendons, ligaments, and joints in the injured area, telling them *not* to move to allow the area to recover and heal. However, the back is a region of the body that gets used every day because you need to keep moving around. If this movement affects the injured area of the spine, another 'ouch' message is sent to the brain, and the brain responds again, saying, 'Don't move.'

As you live and need to move, this cycle continues. The brain increases the sensitivity in this area to prevent pain and movement. Over time, the muscles become extremely tight and weak because of lack of use, joints stiffen up, and the fluidity of the joint is lost as the synovial fluid thickens. Any time this area moves, the pain triggers, and it starts a cycle (negative feedback) from the spine to the brain and the brain to the muscles.

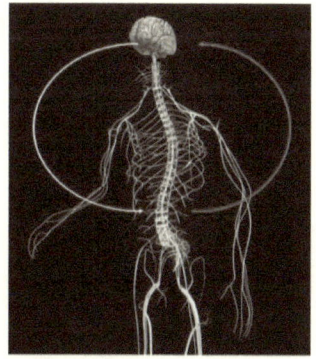

Figure 14. *Continually moving leads to this message loop – 'ouch' and 'don't move'.*

The problem with this situation is you need to break the negative feedback loop to allow the hypersensitivity to return to normal in order to reduce pain. The most natural way to break this negative feedback loop is exercise. Exercise releases endorphins (happy hormones), which makes us feel good, reducing the pain.

The parasympathetic and the sympathetic nervous systems are like a seesaw; when one is on, the other is off. Therefore by turning on the parasympathetic nervous system, you turn off the nervous system that drives pain. Therefore there should be, and there is, a reduction in the neurological processes that cause pain, allowing the pain level to subside.

Click the link below or scan the code to learn more
about understanding chronic back pain
https://www.stopbackpain.com.au/stop-back-pain-turn-off-the-pain

ACTIVITY: HOW DO WE TURN OFF THE PAIN?

YOU NEED TO reduce stress. This is incredibly hard when you are in pain and unable to function normally in everyday life. But when doing these exercises, you need to try to switch off your stress and find a relaxed state. Here are the top four exercises I specifically use to reduce pain and activate the parasympathetic nervous system.

TVA breathing. Breathing is one of the simplest activities we do in life. Yet so many people breathe incorrectly. The correct technique is termed 'diaphragmatic breathing'. As you breathe in, your stomach should push out first, and then your chest should expand. A lot of people only breathe from their chest. You can see this in more detail on our *Back Pain Eliminator* DVD series.

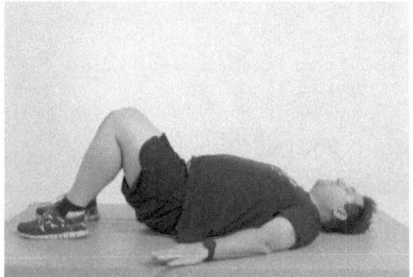 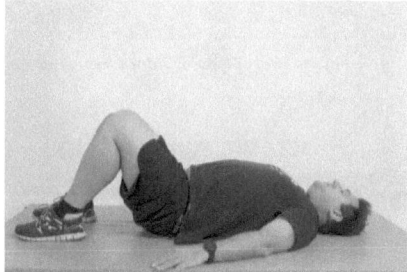

Figure 15. TVA breathing assists in reducing the pain.

1. Lie on your back with your knees bent.
2. Push out your stomach as though it's bloated.
3. Take a deep breath.
4. As you breathe out, draw your stomach in.
5. Push out your stomach as you breathe in; draw your stomach in as you breathe out.

TVA four-point stance (decompression). This is my go-to exercise to help people reduce back pain. By just placing yourself in this position, it will help reduce your pain. Most importantly, ensure you're in a quiet environment; don't have kids jumping on you or other distractions. Then you can focus on your breathing while doing this exercise. Kneeling on the floor on all fours, try to develop what's termed a 'neutral spine'.

Attempt to develop a neutral spine. (You might need a mirror.) Become familiar with the position of each part of your body so you can repeat it whenever needed.

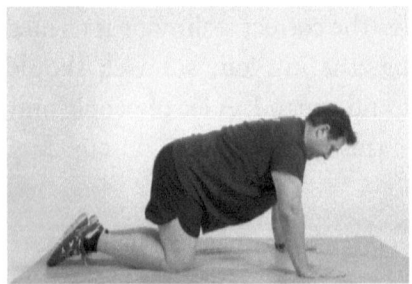 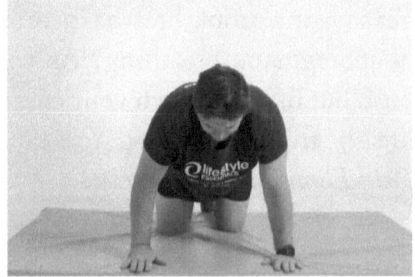

Figure 16. Four-point stance helps reduce pain via the parasympathetic nervous system.

1. Activate your TVA by drawing in your abdomen.
2. Take the weight out of the opposite arm and leg, but keep the hand and knee in contact with the floor.
3. Alternate from one side to the other, taking the weight out of the opposite arm and leg.
4. Try not to let the hips rotate or move; keep them straight and still.

Vertical foam roller. This exercise helps turn on your parasympathetic nervous system. By lying on the roller lengthwise, it opens up the chest, increasing your lung capacity. This helps you breathe easier, which in turn relaxes the body and stimulates the parasympathetic nervous system.

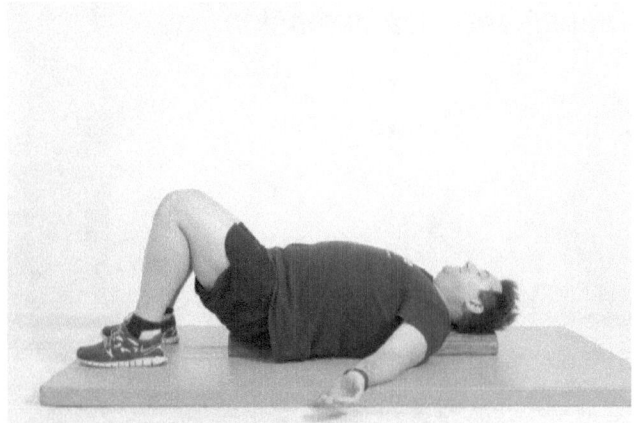

Figure 17. Vertical foam roller assists in stretching the chest and reducing pain.

1. Find a quiet environment to do this exercise.
2. Place the roller on the floor or on a mat. Ensure it's on a flat surface and can't move.
3. Lie on the roller so both your head and tail bone are on the roller.
4. Once on the roller, place your arms on the floor.
5. Take slow, deep breaths, ideally using diaphragmatic breathing – stomach rises before the chest.

Neural mobilisation leg extension.

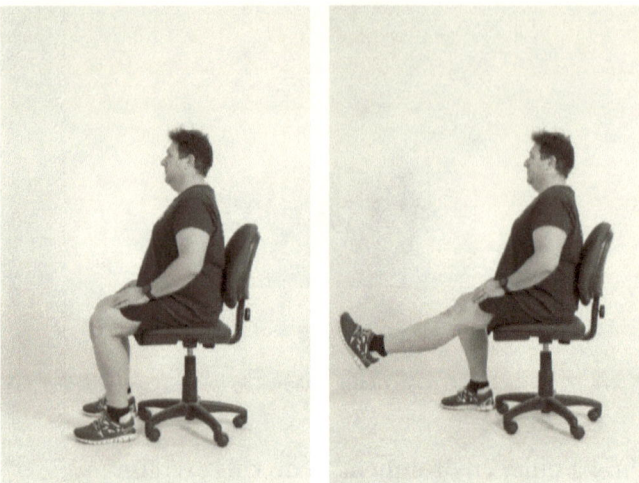

Figure 18. Neural mobilisation assists in desensitising the pain.

1. Sit up straight on a chair (like a piece of string is pulling you up to the ceiling) with your feet flat on the floor.
2. Keep sitting upright, and slowly extend your leg. (Make sure this is slow and only as far as you can go without causing pain in your back; pulling is OK.)
3. Return the foot to the floor.

EFFECTS OF LONG-TERM CHRONIC PAIN

ONE OF THE other major effects of being in chronic pain is the shortening of the nervous system. It doesn't actually shorten, but it does send a message to the muscles that it has shortened. As shown in the negative feedback loop, the brain will try to stop the body from moving when it's in pain. It does this on a number of levels. Firstly, it will increase the pain receptors' sensitivity in an attempt to stop you from moving. Secondly, the brain will cause the muscles to contract, therefore shortening them, trying to stop the body from moving. This will cause other consequences such as joint stiffness and loss in mobility.

The next issue is where the brain starts to communicate that the nervous system has shortened. For example, somebody in chronic back pain will often lose flexibility and be unable to touch their toes.

The body is simply doing everything it can to stop the painful area from moving. It first does it by creating pain; then it makes the muscles tight so that they can't move. Next, it stiffens the joints; and finally, it communicates that the body has lost the neurological ability to overstretch. When you're in the neurologically shortened state and overstretch (or are overstretched by a therapist or a trainer), it can cause the body to go into neural shock. This will cause a massive increase in pain and the intensity of the whole cycle. When you're in this cycle, the pain should be turned off, but the nervous system also needs to be mobilised to prevent this ongoing cycle.

Neural Mobilisation Exercises

By doing each of these four exercises – TVA breathing, four-point stance, leg extension mobilisation, and vertical foam roller – the parasympathetic nervous system will turn off the pain mechanisms.

Then the neural mobilisation will give the neurological system the opportunity to return to its normal state and stop triggering such a hypersensitive pain response.

Posture

When dealing with poor or incorrect posture, it's often asked, 'Do tight muscles cause poor posture?' or 'Does poor posture cause tight muscles?' The answer is yes – it's a chicken-or-egg scenario. Placing your body continually into poor or incorrect postures will cause the muscles to shorten, but when you hurt or injure a muscle, it will shorten; and if this occurs for a prolonged period, this will also affect a person's posture. In helping people overcome back pain, it's essential that both muscle tightness and incorrect posture are dealt with together.

The majority of back pain will start with either an injury or incorrect loading through the spine. Injuries can cause a direct problem such as a prolapsed disc, a bulge, or a fracture. Incorrect loading is more likely to lead to nerve impingement, muscle tightness, and mobility issues. In discussing such a huge area, I would break it down by condition. Each of these sections will give you a basic understanding of the condition and how it could be treated.

Back Conditions (Injuries)

With disc injuries, people will often say, 'I have put my back out,' or use the term 'slipped disc' to describe an injury. The interesting part is when you ask them what they mean, they often don't know. This section will define the difference between these different injuries and help you seek the correct treatment.

Waiver: In clinical practice, I will never diagnose or allow a person to self-diagnose a disc injury or any type of dysfunction without a medical scan. If a person reports they have a bulged disc, unless there's a scan showing a bulge, don't take this as fact. There's no such thing as a practitioner with X-ray vision who can do what an MRI can do. If you have chronic pain and you haven't had a medical scan, it's my strong recommendation that you have a scan to rule out any structural problems.

An X-ray will demonstrate a bony structure. It will show fractures on the bone, the shape of the bone (wear and tear), and the overall structural shape of the disc. An MRI will show much greater detail, showing the structure and integrity of the bones, tendons, ligaments, muscles, and intervertebral discs. An MRI is a much better scan for establishing the whole picture.

EXCESSIVE WEAR AND TEAR OF THE SPINE

AS ANY STRUCTURE of the body is subject to stress, it's only normal that there would be a certain amount of wear and tear, and the spine is no exception. The amount of wear and tear on the spine is directly affected by the person's posture. For example, a person who has a good strong posture will have less stress on the vertebral column and, hence, less degeneration on the spine. It's more likely that a person with poor posture will see an increase in the amount of degeneration of the spine.

Figure 7 shows an example of different stages of spinal degeneration. The top vertebra in this picture demonstrates a normal disc. As we age and participate in activities which cause postural changes, incorrect loading on the spine causes degeneration of the vertebrae or the discs. If this type of loading on the spine continues, it can lead to greater problems, such as thinning of the discs, bulging discs, and even a prolapsed disc.

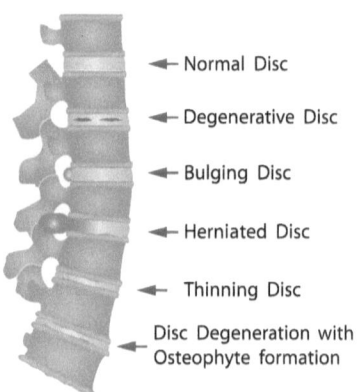

← Normal Disc

← Degenerative Disc

← Bulging Disc

← Herniated Disc

← Thinning Disc

← Disc Degeneration with Osteophyte formation

Figure 19. Degeneration of the spine.

Please note that degeneration of the spine has become very common in today's society, and in the majority of cases, you *don't need to undergo a surgical procedure.* If a specialist recommends that you need surgery for any spinal problem, please explore all avenues before you do so.

Disc Bulge

A disc bulge is a condition that needs to be taken extremely seriously. A bulged disc is only one step away from permanent damage – a prolapsed disc. Most disc bulges occur in the lower back (lumbar region) because it's the weight-bearing region of the spine.

When a person has incorrect posture such as an excessive curve in their spine or excessive lordosis, then this pressure is transferred to the disc in the form of incorrect loading. This force applied to the disc can cause it to bulge either forwards or backwards. If this pressure continues to force the disc outwards, it weakens the wall of the disc, which can lead to either a tear or loss of strength, allowing it to bulge out of shape.

When a bulged disc protrudes backwards, it reduces the space in the spinal canal. If the bulge is large enough, it will irritate the spinal cord, causing symptoms such as numbness and tingling in the legs or feet, sciatic pain, muscle weakness, and constant debilitating pain. This ongoing pain can lead to the symptoms spoken about in earlier chapters, with a negative feedback loop and even neural shortening.

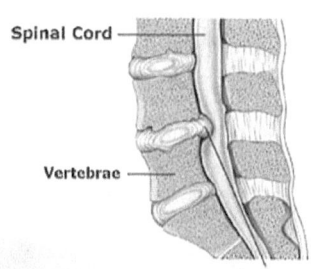

Figure 20. Disc bulge.

Prolapsed Disc

A prolapsed disc is when the wall of the intervertebral disc ruptures, allowing the contents of the disc to spill out into the tunnel that houses the spinal cord (figure 8). Once the integrity of the intervertebral disc has gone, the bones will often collapse, irritating and even trapping nerves, thereby causing pain, numbness, sciatica, and other types of dysfunctions.

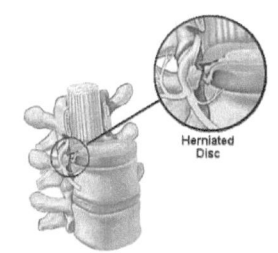

Figure 21. A disc bugle can often develop into a prolapsed disc.

Once a prolapsed disc has occurred, there's nothing an allied health professional can do to return the disc to normal. To have the disc fixed, you'll need to look at surgical options. However, with any spinal surgery, make sure you investigate this thoroughly as people can often end up in more pain after having spinal surgery than before.

One of the major ongoing problems for a person with a prolapsed disc is that the injured section of the spine no longer moves correctly. This is why it will often be suggested that a spinal fusion be carried out. However, the problem is that once the spine is fused together, it can't move at all. This means that the sections of the spine above and below this area need to compensate for the fused segment. This will often lead to more dysfunctions of the discs above and below the fusion and even further injury.

You can't live with pain from a prolapsed disc. By desensitising the nervous system and strengthening the core muscles and the lower back muscles through the core, the muscles can, and will, reduce the pressure and load on the injured area, reducing the pain. By strengthening the muscles of the spine, you'll also prevent the likelihood of further injuries due to immobility of the injured area.

Spondylolisthesis (A Slipped Disc)

Most people use the term 'slipped disc' to describe a bulge or a prolapsed disc. A true slipped disc is known as spondylolisthesis. This is where part of (or the entire) vertebra slips forwards onto the vertebra (figure 9). This is a structural condition that can't be adjusted or fixed without surgical intervention. This can lead to chronic

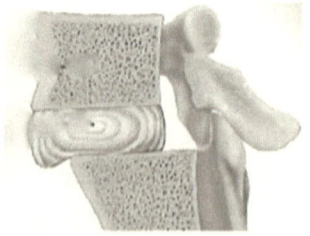

Figure 22. A slipped disc is when the vertebra moves forwards as shown above.

back pain and nerve impingement. However, by strengthening the lower back, a person can live pain-free with such a condition.

Sacroiliac Joint Dysfunction

This joint connects the vertebral column (base of the spine) to the pelvis.

The primary function of the sacroiliac (SI) joint is shock absorption, helping distribute the weight of the body up the spine. The sacroiliac joint is a slightly moveable joint, only allowing 2–4 mm of movement. When this joint is not functioning correctly, it loses its ability to move, becoming stiff and 'locked'. This type of dysfunction can lead to muscle imbalances, nerve impingement, osteopubitis, and uneven leg length discrepancies. Furthermore, it loses its ability to provide shock absorption for the spine, causing further increased spinal stress.

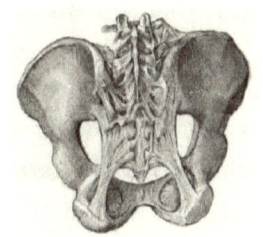

Figure 23. The sacrum forms a joint with the pelvis, known as the sacroiliac joint.

Uneven Leg length

There are two types of uneven leg length, functional and structural. A structural discrepancy is when one of the leg bones is longer than the other. The only way to accurately diagnosis this is by a 1:1 X-ray, which is then measured by a tape measure. Functional discrepancies are where something happens in the body, such as spinal curve or muscle tightness, which leads to a difference in the leg length. However, the bones are the same length.

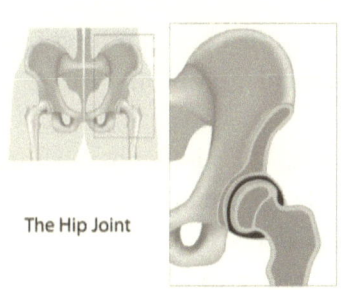

The Hip Joint

Figure 24. How the hip bone sits in the pelvis affects the leg length.

The hip joint is a ball-and-socket synovial joint. This means the joint is freely moveable. In relation to leg length, the position of the head of the femur (leg bone) can affect the length of the leg. You can see in the picture that if one of the hip joints was jarred into the pelvis and the other was loose, it would affect the length of the pelvis height and, in turn, the leg length.

When there's a difference in leg length, it will cause changes in the person's pelvis, tilting it forwards or backwards or elevating one side. Overall, these changes in the pelvis will carry through into the spine and create abnormal curves.

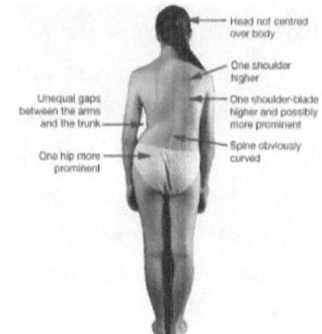

Figure 25. Uneven leg length will affect the whole body.

Stress Fractures

When people hear that someone has broken their back, they often ask if they're paralysed. There's a big difference between a broken bone in the vertebral column and spinal cord damage. A person can fracture their spine (vertebra) without damaging the spinal cord.

The vertebra will tend to fracture in three areas: the vertebral body, the arch, and the part of the spine that protrudes the back of the vertebra.

A fractured spine can cause back pain as there are numerous pain receptors in your bones. Once you've had a scan to diagnose your problem, please spend some time with a good allied health professional who has experience at dealing with this particular problem.

A fracture will heal because bones are alive, and although you may not continue to grow taller, new bones are laid down every seven years throughout your life. The more stress (physical load) you place on your bones, the stronger they become. The best way to strengthen your bones and prevent fractures and other bone-related diseases, such as osteoporosis, is to participate in a regular resistance training program (not by drinking milk).

Please note that just because a person is a *qualified* health professional, it doesn't mean they're a *good* health professional, nor does it mean they're active in continuous self-improvement.

No matter what type of doctor or allied health professional you see, it's never wrong to get a second opinion if you're uncomfortable or unsure about what the first health professional is saying.

I always recommend that people should understand not only what the practitioner is saying but also why they're doing what they're doing. When it comes to surgical procedures on the spine, make sure you have explored all other alternative therapies *first*.

Compressed Nerves

The spinal cord forms a blueprint of the body (dermatomes). As nerves come off the spinal cord, they travel through small channels in the vertebra. If these small channels become blocked, it can compress or impinge the nerve. It can be either inhibited or stimulated, leading to muscles not working correctly and pain receptors becoming more sensitive to movement. Continual impingement of the nerves can lead to pain, numbness, muscle weakness, muscle fatigue, muscle tightness, or even pins and needles in this specific part of the body. Certain areas of the spine will affect body functions such as gastrointestinal, respiratory, and cardiac functions.

USE YOUR CORE

'USE YOUR CORE.' This is one of the most overused statements in relation to back pain, with allied health and medical professionals often stating that you need to strengthen your core or you need to do 'clinical Pilates'. A lot of the time, this is correct. You do need to strengthen your core; but first, you must learn how to use your core correctly. Don't just 'use it'. The problem (when it comes to back pain) is that if you're not using your core properly, it won't support your back.

Like other parts of the body, if you don't use and enhance your core muscles and use them correctly, the TVA will weaken or lose its neural connection and stop working.

Why Is the Core So Important?

The core is the group of muscles that form the bridge between the spine, the spinal muscles, and your abdominals. However, having a six-pack is not part of having a strong core. A six-pack is related to the composition of body fat, not the ability to correctly activate your core, although being excessively overweight will prevent you from activating your core.

To have a strong back, you must have strong abdominal muscles. But this doesn't mean you'll have a strong back. Preventing back pain depends on correctly activating your abdominals, not just the strength of the muscles.

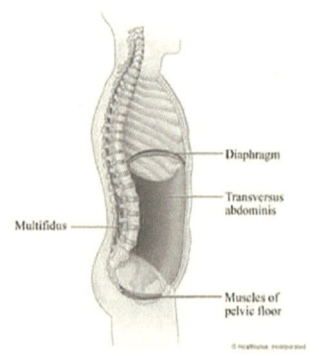

Figure 26. The muscles that make up the inner unit.

Your core can be broken up into an inner unit and an outer unit. The inner unit is essential for stabilising the spine and forming the foundation of the movement for the pelvis and spine. The inner unit is composed of the transverse abdominis, pelvic floor, diaphragm, and multifidus.

The outer unit is composed of larger muscles and is used in gross movements such as bending. The outer unit is composed of many different muscles including the rectus abdominis, the obliques, and the larger erector spinae muscles.

Activation of your core will reduce and may even eliminate back pain by transferring pressure from the spine and surrounding muscles into the abdominals. However, the key to using your core in the prevention of back pain is learning how to activate your inner unit independently to the outer unit. If you can't do this, it's likely that the inner unit won't work in combination with the outer unit, thereby leaving the spine unstable.

Understanding the Inner Unit

The inner unit is composed of four different muscles that all work together to stabilise the spine. The TVA, diaphragm, pelvic floor, and the multifidus (one of the deep erector spinae muscles) form a cube like support network for the pelvis, ribs, and lower back.

All the inner unit muscles work together to support and stabilise the spine, but each has a specific function in the body. The pelvic floor forms the support in the pelvis. It aids in bladder control but also has a connection with the TVA to form a co-activation. When you contract the pelvic floor, you also see a co-activation of the TVA. This means that you can activate your TVA through the pelvic floor, which doesn't affect breathing.

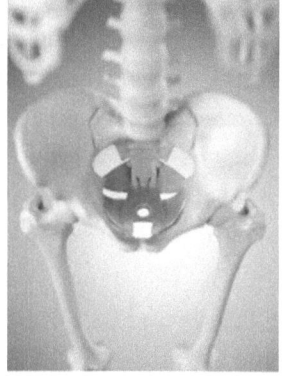

Figure 27. The pelvic floor.

The multifidus is a deep muscle that forms part of the erector spinae group. This is a segmental muscle involved in stabilising and rotating the spine at individual levels. The multifidus is responsible for directly supporting the spine, connecting one vertebra to the next. It helps with segmental rotation so that each individual vertebra is moving correctly. This means when the spine rotates as a whole, the individual vertebra is moving correctly and is supported.

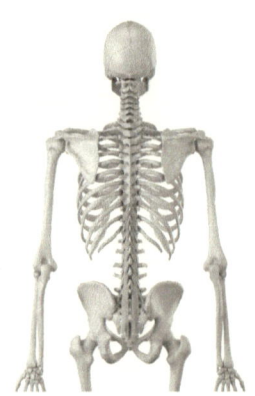

Figure 28. The multifidus.

The diaphragm connects your inner unit to the respiratory system, thereby ensuring that correct breathing patterns are occurring within the body. Your respiration is one of the most essential components of being healthy. It delivers oxygen to your muscles so they can function correctly. Correct breathing also ensures the stomach muscles support the spine. Breathing correctly is a rhythmic pattern. As you breathe in, the stomach rises first, and then the chest expands, allowing the TVA to support the stomach. The rising of the stomach creates room in the abdominal cavity. This concept of space neurologically allows the TVA to contract, which then supports the lower back.

When the breathing pattern is incorrect, it will often lead to either thoracic breathing (from the chest) or abdominal breathing (from the stomach). This has several effects on the body. Firstly, it decreases lung capacity, reducing the body's oxygen levels, creating a negative impact on the muscles' ability to function correctly. Secondly, the incorrect breathing pattern prevents the TVA from functioning correctly to support the spine. That's why it's essential that you learn to breathe correctly and turn your core on through the pelvic floor rather than the stomach.

One of the more commonly known muscles of the inner unit is the transverse abdominis (also known as the TVA). This is the deepest abdominal muscle which wraps around the body like a belt, connecting the back muscles (erector spinae) to the abdominal region via the thoracolumbar fascia. By doing this, the TVA can transfer pressure from the back into the abdominal regions, reducing the pressure in the spine.

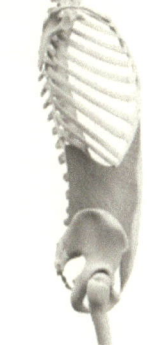

Figure 29. Transversus abdominis.

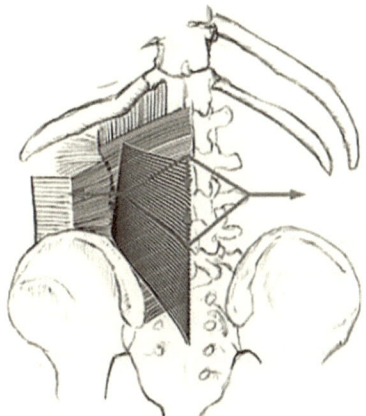

Figure 30. TVA attaches into the connective tissue in the lower back, which transfers pressure out of the back into the abdominals.

Transverse Abdominis Weight Belt Action

The TVA is joined to a connective tissue wrapped around the back muscles (thoracolumbar fascia). When the TVA activates, it causes a co-activation of the erector spinae muscles, which aids in the transfer of pressure from the spinal muscles supporting the back into the abdominal muscles. This reduces the direct load on the spine and the intervertebral discs.

When the TVA doesn't work correctly, the back muscles need to work harder to stabilise and move the spine. Furthermore, this makes other abdominal muscles, such as the rectus abdominis and the obliques, try to support the spine. However, the function of these muscles is bending the spine forwards and rotating the spine, not stabilising it. This all means the spine moves without stable foundations, which can weaken the deep spinal muscles and the intervertebral discs, increasing the likelihood of injury or postural dysfunction.

Supporting the inner unit muscles are the outer unit muscles. This is composed of the muscle that wraps around the outside of the torso, the rectus abdominis (six-pack muscle), the internal and external obliques, and the larger back muscles. These muscles help support movements of the body that are too heavy for the inner unit to handle. More information will be covered about the outer unit in later chapters on muscle slings.

The inner unit and the outer unit work as a team. The inner unit sets the foundation for the pelvis and spine so the outer unit has a firm structure to work off. If one isn't working correctly (usually the inner unit), this will weaken the body and, in turn, the person's posture, which can lead to injury or postural weaknesses.

In a rehabilitation program, it's essential to start with the inner unit. Get this activated independently first. Then integrate with the outer unit correctly. In many cases, it doesn't, which means that when a person lifts a heavy weight, there's no support for the foundation of the pelvis or spine and no communication between the deep spinal muscles and the abdominal muscles.

How to Use Your Core

One of the most effective ways of teaching people how to use their core is through activating their pelvic floor. By engaging your pelvic floor, you activate your deep abdominal muscles (TVA). One of the most effective ways to activate your pelvic floor is to use your muscle as though you're attempting to prevent yourself from going to the toilet. This activation of the pelvic floor co-activates the deep abdominal muscles. By using this co-activation technique to strengthen your pelvic floor, you also strengthen your TVA. In addition to this, you also strengthen the connection between the TVA and pelvic floor, which is essential for being able to turn on your core while breathing.

Isolating Your Core

The following exercise is specifically designed to strengthen the activation between your pelvic floor and TVA without affecting your breathing. These exercises allow you to isolate the pelvic floor and TVA without the outer unit muscles switching on.

The important aspect of these exercises is to maintain diaphragmatic breathing because it's essential for the correct activation of the TVA.

Pelvic Floor and TVA Activation

<u>Click her to learn how to active your TVA via your pelvic floor</u>
<u>https://www.stopbackpain.com.au/stop-back-pain-pelvic-floor</u>

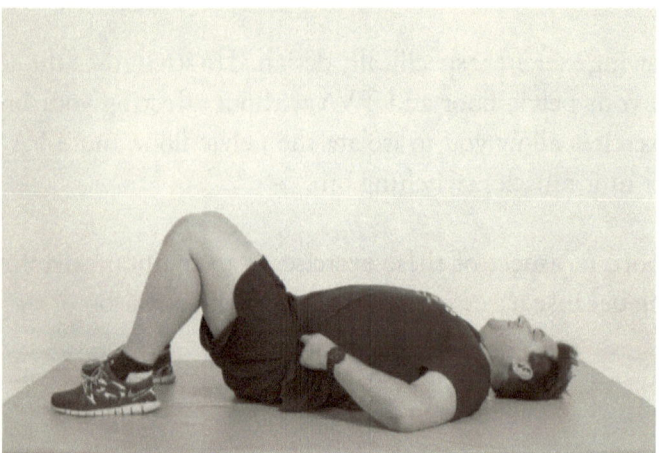

Figure 31. Activating the pelvic floor will activate the TVA, reducing back pain.

1. Lie on your back in a quiet, relaxed setting.
2. Place your hands on the inside of the front bony part of your hips.
3. Turn on your pelvic floor by internally preventing yourself from going to the bathroom.
4. Under your fingers you should feel a taut band pulling on each side of the hips – this is your TVA.
5. Continue to turn on your pelvic floor for about five seconds, off and on for another five seconds, and then off.
6. Repeat this 15–20 times.

You can also do this exercise while sitting in the car every time you stop at a red light or when you go to the bathroom.

Pelvic Floor and TVA Heel Taps

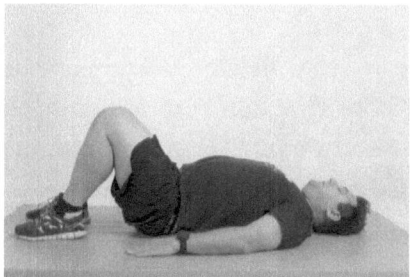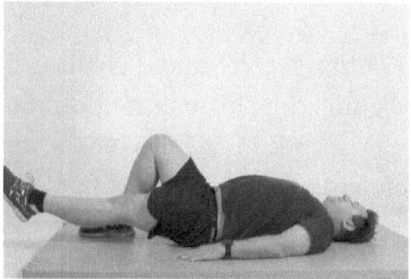

Figure 32. Activating the TVA while extending the leg will increase the load on the lower back, strengthening the abdominals.

1. Lie on your back with your knees bent in a quiet, relaxed setting. Keep diaphragmatically breathing the whole time.
2. Place your hands on the inside of the front bony part of your hips.
3. Turn on your pelvic floor by internally preventing yourself from going to the bathroom.
4. Under your fingers, you should feel a taut band pulling on each side of the hips – this is your TVA.
5. Try to keep your pelvic floor turned on the whole time.
6. Slowly lift one leg off the floor and extend it out straight, touch the heel on the floor, and then return the foot to the starting position.
7. Repeat on the other side, keeping the pelvic floor on the whole time.
8. Continue to alternate sides, attempting to keep the TVA active through the pelvic floor.

USE IT OR LOSE IT

WHEN WE USE and challenge our muscles, they grow and increase the functional strength of our body. When we don't use our muscles, they shrink in size, becoming weaker and weaker. This has a number of negative effects on the body. One of the most essential components to any healthy lifestyle is resistance training.

Dysfunction will often occur when you don't keep the body strong and when you ignore the body by becoming sedentary as seen in the following example.

> Roger, a 78-year-old man, walked into our personal training studio in 2005. When I asked him to sit down on the couch and have a chat about how we can help, he said, 'If I sit down there, I will never get up.' After a lengthy chat, Roger told me how he was struggling to get out of bed; simple activities such as standing up or sitting down in a chair had become difficult tasks. This is not uncommon; you observe older people having difficulty sitting down in lower chairs and then requiring assistance to get up.

This is a perfect example of the theory 'use it or lose it'.

When you don't use muscles, they waste away, and this is known as atrophy. As muscles become weaker, it becomes more difficult to function and do normal everyday activities such as sitting down and standing up. Unfortunately, this process of atrophy is normal and will naturally start to occur after the age of 20 years. It can have devastating effects on the body, with the average sedentary person losing about 200–400 grams of muscle every year. This has a number of negative effects on the body such as the following:

- a decrease in energy levels
- a decrease in metabolism

- an increase in stress and load in the joints
- an increase in joint pain and joint stiffness
- a reduction in range of movement
- a reduction in strength
- a reduction in fat burning
- weakening connective tissues such as tendons and ligaments

In relation to the spine, this loss in muscle mass can lead to an increase in pain. As the muscles that support the spine weaken, so do the connective tissue, tendons, ligaments, and joint capsule. Over time, this increased pressure on the joints of the spine will lead to joint pain.

Other muscles start to compensate for these weaknesses in the body, leading to further dysfunction. In the spine, there are muscles that move the vertebra, and other muscles help stabilise and support it. As muscle weakens due to a sedentary lifestyle, the ability to move, stabilise, and support the spine is reduced. These weaker muscles are unable to transfer pressure out of the vertebral joints into the muscles. Hence more pressure is now carried directly in the joint, and this increase leads to a greater amount of wear and tear (degeneration) on the vertebral joints and surrounding structures. The only way to prevent this from occurring or reverse this effect is to strengthen the muscles.

There are twenty-four different joints that make up the vertebral column, and they're all stabilised by a group of muscles called the erector spinae. If this muscle group atrophies, their ability to support the spine is diminished. The major weight-bearing portion of the spine is the lower back, known as the lumbar spine. If the muscles in this region are unable to support the weight-bearing function of the spine, it will lead to pain and dysfunction.

The erector spinae is responsible for moving, supporting, and stabilising the spine. Ultimately, its role is to help transfer the load out of the spine into the abdominals, thereby reducing pressure on the spine.

The erector spinae is classified into two groups, a superficial group and a deep group. The deep erector spinae muscles are specifically designed to do segmental movement (movement across individual vertebrae – one segment at a time). These form a lattice-type support network across the joint, helping transfer pressure out of the joint.

Functionally, these muscles segmentally stabilise and rotate the individual vertebra. When they're unable to support the spine effectively due to a weakness, injury, or dysfunction, there's an increased load placed on the vertebral joints and the intervertebral disc. This can cause joint stiffness, loss of mobility, and degeneration of the spine. Overall, the spine loses its ability to move and stabilise at a segmental level, which in turn leads to a decrease in a person's range of movement and to trapped nerves and other structural problems.

The superficial spinal muscles extend from either side of the pelvis to a few different levels of the spine and the ribs. These muscles aid in the stabilisation of the spine but are the prime movers in bending backwards and sideways. The superficial erector spinae forms an outer brace across the spine, helping support the deeper segmental muscles. The outer muscles also link with the deep abdominal muscles, allowing a connection between the spinal muscles and abdominals, helping transfer the load out of the back and the spine into the abdominal muscles. Therefore using your abdominals correctly is essential in developing a strong back.

Muscles Always Remain Taut!

Muscles work in pairs; this relationship is called an agonist and antagonist pairing. As one muscle shortens, another muscle will lengthen. An example

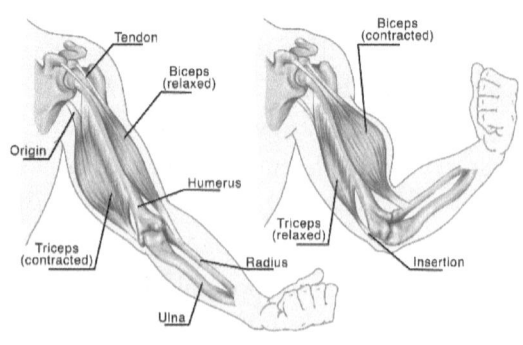

Figure 33. Muscles work in teams.

of this is your arm muscles. When you bend your elbow, the muscle in the front of your arm (biceps muscle) shortens (agonist). For this to occur, the muscle in the back of the arm (triceps) relaxes and lengthens (antagonist). When your back muscles are tight, other muscles in the hips and abdominals will lengthen. If muscles remain in this lengthened position for a prolonged period, they'll become weaker, leading to a greater imbalance in the body and an increase likelihood of pain and dysfunction.

Being contractile tissues, they always remain taut, whether in a lengthened or shortened position of contraction. When a muscle contracts concentrically, it shortens. When this occurs, the filaments sliding over each other (overlapping) bring the two ends of the muscle closer together, unlike a rope, which goes loose as you bring the two ends together.

When a muscle contracts eccentrically or lengthens, these filaments slide out, so there's less overlap, and the ends of the muscle move away from each other. This sliding mechanism is known as the sliding filament theory.

The strength of a muscle is dependent on the amount of overlap. A muscle will be at its strongest point when it's at the midpoint of contraction. It has a large amount of overlap and can continue to generate movement. A muscle is at its weakest point when the muscle is fully extended (little overlap) or fully contracted (completely overlapped). It's weak at both points of the contraction because the muscle can't generate a strong contraction. From a practical sense, this means a person's muscles are at their weakest point when fully elongated or fully contracted, which is the end of their movement.

Understand that when a muscle becomes weaker, there's an increased amount of pressure on the joint. It's easy to see how a basic sedentary lifestyle, which does cause a decrease in muscle mass and strength, can increase the likelihood of back pain, especially in the weight-bearing region of the lower back.

Muscles Play Different Roles

A muscle can play different roles, each being dependent on the movement that is occurring. A muscle will functionally do one of three roles: move the joint (agonist), relax so that the joint can move (antagonist), or stabilise the joint so that it can move safely. The role in which a specific muscle will undertake is totally dependent on the movement that is occurring.

An example of this is the erector spinae muscle, which will act as an agonist when bending backwards. However, these same muscles relax and lengthen when the spine bends forwards. In other movements, such as lifting or walking, these same muscles stabilise the spine so it remains strong and forms a solid foundation for the movement.

When a muscle is injured or overused, it's unable to react normally by shortening to protect itself and the joint from further damage. If this muscle is left untreated for prolonged periods, the body will reprogram the muscle to believe that this shortened new length of the muscle is normal. Once this reprogramming has occurred, the joint will adapt to the new length, leading to a loss of mobility and full range of movement. This is often seen in the hamstrings; when a person has lower back pain, they often lose flexibility in their hamstrings. (They can't touch their toes.) This often occurs because the brain doesn't want the nervous system to be overstretched. The most effective way to avoid this is to prevent the muscle from moving.

When this happens in the spinal muscles, from an injury or postural change, it will stop the vertebra column from being able to move correctly. Hence there's a loss of mobility in a section of the spine, and this is reflected in other areas of the spine that try to overcompensate for the lack of movement in one area with a greater amount of movement in another area. Eventually, this will lead to further imbalances in the loading of the spine, which can cause disc problems, trapped nerves, and other forms of dysfunction and pain.

In summing up, your muscular system is designed to support and move your body. Unfortunately, if you don't use your muscles, they'll become weaker. This has numerous negative effects on the body. All of these effects can be avoided by simply moving. By participating in regular exercise, plus specific strength training exercises, you'll prevent atrophy.

What should I do?

1. Participate in a functional strength training program at least once or twice a week to prevent muscle atrophy.
2. Move more. Look for opportunities to move more often throughout your day (walking to work, taking the stairs, playing sport).
3. Stretching is an essential part of any exercise program. Look at stretching your major muscles as often as possible.

Get Your Butt Working

Your butt muscles (gluteal muscles) play a vital role in your body's ability to function without back pain. The major role of the gluteal muscles is to help extend the hip and stabilise the hip joint. Extension of the hip is the movement that occurs at the hip when a person stands up from the seated position. Another role of the gluteal muscles is stabilisation of the hip joint. This is the joint where the femur (leg bone) connects to the pelvis (at the acetabulum). This can lead to problems with pelvic stability and the sacroiliac joint and an uneven leg length, all of which are related to back pain.

Unfortunately, the gluteal muscles can stop functioning correctly. This will have many side effects in your posture, specifically in the hip and lower back. This phenomenon of the glutes not working is due to a loss of neural awareness, which can occur because of too much sitting.

Muscles are connected to the brain via neural pathways, better described as the body's electrical wiring. This is seen when we do activities that require higher levels of coordination. The first time you do the activity, you lack coordination, and it's more difficult. But as you repeat the activity, you develop neurological pathways that allow you to better coordinate the movement. The more you do the activity, the more automated the movement and behaviour becomes.

In today's society, we spend about 50–90 per cent of our day sitting. This has led to an increase in the incidence of people not correctly activating their gluteus muscles correctly. When these muscles don't work correctly, your lower back and hamstrings work harder to compensate for this latent muscle. Thinking of this as a train, there are three carriages: the back muscles, the gluteal muscles, and the hamstrings. When the gluteal muscles stop working, the other two carriages are required to compensate, which increases the functional load on the back and the hamstrings. Over time, this increase in load will lead to dysfunction in either one or both of the compensating muscles. The muscle that's most affected is dependent on the movements and activities the person does.

A person who is more sedentary will usually have more issues in the lower back, while athletes or people who lead active lifestyles tend to have more issues in their hamstrings.

Michael Clarke, the Australian cricketer, is well known for having back issues. Over time, he also generated hamstring issues, which often occur hand in hand. In the end, these injuries ended his cricket career. It begs the question 'did his glutes work?'

Getting Your Butt Working

The first step to getting a muscle working correctly is to neurologically reconnect the muscle with the brain. When you palpate a muscle, you raise the neurological awareness of that muscle with the brain. This is one way to get the muscle to start working more efficiently. Similarly, an effective way to neurologically reconnect a muscle through exercises is to isolate the muscle by using it on its own.

Unfortunately, a lot of people use compound exercises, such as squats and lunges, to try to strengthen the gluteal muscles. However, if the gluteal muscles aren't working independently, they won't work correctly as a team, which is required in an exercise such as a squat.

To get a muscle working, we need to first isolate it. Once the muscle has been isolated and is working on its own, it needs to be integrated back into a movement pattern with its team of muscles. Muscles work in functional units – the functional units that extend the hips are the glutes and hamstrings. It's when one or more muscles in a unit stop working that imbalances occur.

By isolating the gluteal muscles, the hip becomes more stable, and you're less likely to suffer from back pain due to pelvic instability.

How to Reconnect Your Glutes

Make sure your backside is working correctly with your back muscles and hamstrings.

Isolated Glute Activation

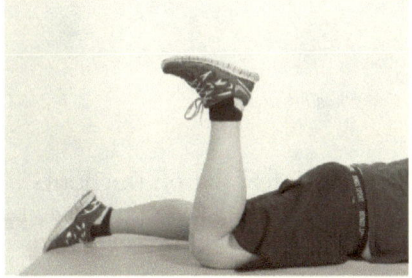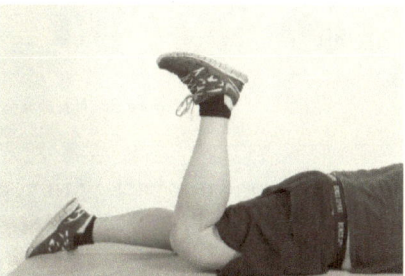

Figure 34. Activating the glutes is essential in strengthening the lower back.

1. Lay on your stomach.
2. Bend one knee ninety degrees.
3. Squeeze your butt tight.
4. Lift your leg off the floor 2–3 cm.

5. Lower your leg back down to the floor.
6. Relax butt muscles.
7. Squeeze your butt tight.
8. Lift leg off floor 2–3 cm.
9. Lower your leg to the floor.
10. Relax butt. Repeat 10–12 times per leg.

More of these videos and exercises can be obtained through www.
stopbackpain.com.au/stop-back-pain-exercise-videos

Integrate your glutes. Once you have isolated your glutes and they're
effectively working in the correct firing sequence, you need to integrate
them back into functional movements with the leg and lower back. The
first step to doing this is with a hip extension.

Hip Extensions

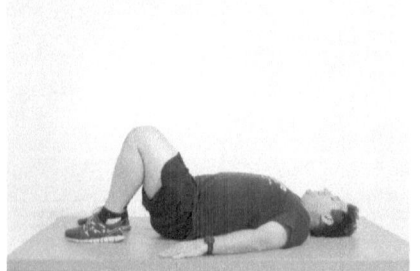 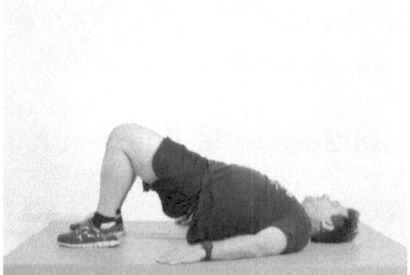

Figure 35. Hip extensions strengthen the glutes.

1. Lie on your back with your knee bent, feet flat on the floor.
2. Activate your pelvic floor, and squeeze your butt muscles like
    you're holding on to a $100 bill.
3. Once everything is activated, lift your hips off the floor (ideally
    to form a straight line from the shoulders to the knees; if you
    can't go this high, start at your own level).
4. Return to the floor and relax, and then repeat from step 2.

Note: Also complete the isolated glute activation before the hip extension as this will ensure the glutes are working correctly and are isolated prior to integrating them into a compound movement. These two exercises are good to do prior to more functional exercises such as squats and lunges as they activate the correct firing sequences.

TEAMWORK

MUSCLES WORK TOGETHER in groups. I refer to these groups as functional units. For example, the inner unit is a functional unit that helps support and stabilise the spine and pelvis.

There are many different functional units in the body. Some always work together as a unit, while others are specifically dependent on the movement that's occurring.

Independently, a muscle can play a number of different roles. When a muscle is doing the work, it's an agonist. If the muscle relaxes and lengthens so the muscle doing the work can shorten, it's an antagonist. Finally, a muscle can be a stabiliser, which supports the joint so other muscles can move the joint correctly (synergist).

An example of this can be seen with the rectus abdominis. Its role as a prime mover is to bend the body forwards. However, it also plays a role in stabilising the trunk when lifting heavy loads and can oppose backward bending but relaxes so the muscle can lengthen as the person bends backwards.

Muscles are commonly looked upon as a single identity. When this happens, treatment and therapy become one-dimensional and are often unsuccessful. However, Thomas Myers developed a concept that all muscles in the body form a network of connections, just like railways. These connections are formed via connective tissues called fascia. This fascia forms a coupling between muscles and is referred to as muscle trains or muscle slings.

Imagine that the muscles in your body are like a train; each individual muscle is a carriage of the train, while the connecting tissue or fascia forms the coupling between the carriages (muscles). When a muscle contracts, this contraction is communicated through all the muscles in that specific sling. Furthermore, the tension created by the contraction and the potential movement of the muscle will transfer through to all the other muscles in that specific train.

Muscle slings work across the whole body, supporting and moving multiple joints to assist the body to move correctly. There are nine specific muscle slings (Myers, 2001), although each sling can affect a person's ability to move, causing the body to compensate, which leads to dysfunction and, in many cases, back pain. We will only discuss specific muscles that are directly related to back pain. If you wish to learn more about muscle trains, I would recommend you read *Anatomy Trains* by Thomas Myers.

In the previous chapter, we discussed the inner and outer units. The key to understanding the outer unit is that there are several of them. The outer unit that's working in partnership with the inner unit is dependent on movement.

For example, the superficial posterior sling works with the inner unit when a person stands upright. It assists in reducing pressure in the spine and ensures a person can develop and maintain strong posture.

Overall, there are seven muscle slings in the body, and they're listed below:

1. *Superficial back line:* runs from the top of your head down your back to the soles of your feet. It forms a connection between the skull and the spinal muscles through to the hamstrings, calves, and feet. The main functional role of this sling is to help keep the body upright.
2. *Superficial front line:* helps balance the body in partnership with the superficial back line. It runs from the tops of the toes up to the pelvis and then connects the abdominals and the thoracic cage to the neck muscles that wrap around the back of the skull.
3. *Lateral line:* the balance line, aiding in balancing the body from front to back as well as left to right. The lateral line aids in the stabilisation of the legs and trunk.

4. *Spiral line:* wraps around the body to support and stabilise movement in all plans. It also aids in rotational movements.
5. *Arm lines:* aid in connecting the arms with the shoulders and major structures in the upper body. There are two arm lines:
   a. deep front line
   b. deep back line
6. *Functional lines:* are rarely used in posture and are used in functional movements such as throwing a ball. The main function of these lines is helping transfer load and movement from one side of the body to the other. There are two functional lines:
   a. back functional line
   b. front functional line
7. *Deep front line:* forms the true core of the body, running from the feet to the skull. It connects the pelvic floor, the lumbar spine, the diaphragm, and the thoracic cage with the skull.

Superficial Posterior Sling

The superficial posterior sling runs down the back of your whole body. It allows communication among your neck, back, hamstring, calf, and foot muscles. When one of these muscles is not functioning correctly, it affects the whole train. Yes, this means that a dysfunctional muscle in your feet may cause back pain or even neck pain.

For the body to function correctly, what first needs to happen is for the inner unit to stabilise the pelvis and spine. The inner unit sets the foundation for the outer movement to move off. Secondly, the outer unit activates to help facilitate and support the movement. This outer unit or sling helps the person standing up straight, such as when going up from a squat or a lunge.

Dysfunction can occur at two levels – at the inner unit level or the outer unit level. If dysfunction occurs at the inner unit level, it causes instability in the spine and pelvis. When this occurs, other muscles (often in the outer unit) will try to stabilise the body. For example, the hamstrings may try to stabilise the pelvic tilt. This will increase the load on the muscles that are trying to stabilise the body, leading to an increased risk of further injuries in these outer muscles.

A client comes in with back pain. They perform a scan, and there's no dysfunction and no pathology to explain the pain. When assessing the client, you establish that the client's TVA is not working. Hence the inner unit is not working. The client has excessive lordosis and an anterior pelvic tilt based on the posture because the inner unit is not stabilising the spine. Other muscles such as the erector spine, hip flexors, and hamstrings are attempting to stabilise the spine, as well as move it. Over time, some of these muscles can become dysfunctional, becoming short and tight or long and weak. This will lead to postural changes, joint stiffness, and other problems related to back pain.

Outer unit dysfunction often occurs from the muscles that are compensating for changes in posture or postural load. When these muscles become dysfunctional (short and tight or long and weak), they can often become injured or cause other issues such as joint stiffness or nerve impingement. When you look at this sling, a person who continually has hamstring issues or tight calves may have some serious health problems.

To ensure that the posterior sling is working correctly, it's essential that the inner unit works. Also, it's important to develop a neutral spine and to ensure the hamstrings are healthy. This can be done by making sure the glutes and hamstrings are working together correctly and that the hamstrings and calves are stretched regularly. By doing this, you'll prevent the posterior sling from becoming dysfunctional.

Stretches for the Posterior Sling

Calf Stretch

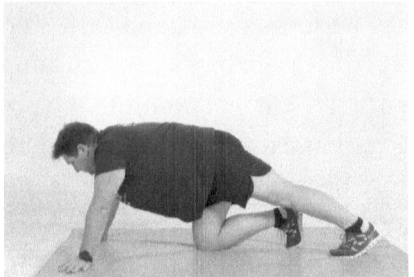

Figure 36. Calf stretch on the floor.

a. Place yourself on your hands and knees; extend one leg back.
b. Pull toe up towards your head and place on the ground.
c. Push back your weight, trying to put the heel down to the floor.

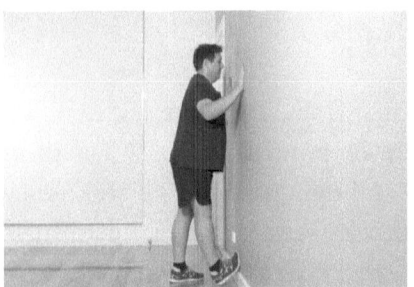

Figure 37. Standing calf stretch.

a. Standing up tall, place your foot against a wall or solid surface, with your toes up towards the ceiling.
b. Push your hips into the wall/pole.
c. Try not to let your heel slip backwards. You should feel a stretch in the calf.

Hamstring Stretch

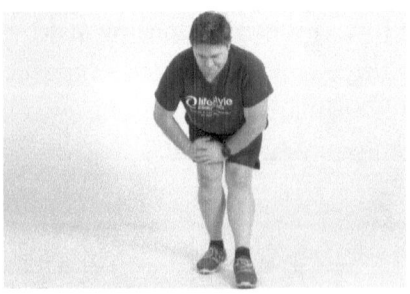

Figure 38. Standing hamstring stretch.

Gluteal Stretches

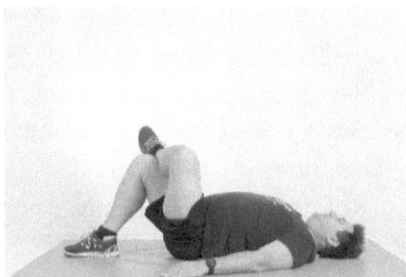

Figure 39. Lying glute stretch start position.

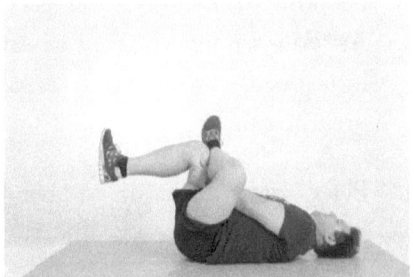

Figure 40. Lying glute stretch – stretching position.

a. Lying on your back with one knee bent, cross the foot over the bent knee.
b. Lift your foot off the floor, grabbing hold of your thigh of the leg lifted off the floor.
c. Pull the leg up to the body.

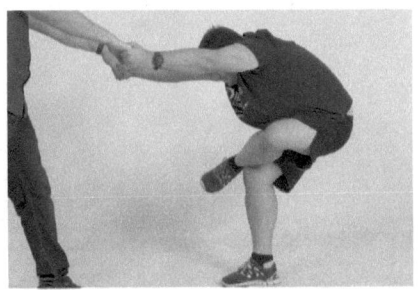

Figure 41. Standing glute stretch.

a. Hold on to a solid support for balance.
b. Cross your leg so your foot is on your opposite knee.
c. Leaning back, bend your knee as you allow yourself to sink backwards. You should feel the stretch in your backside.

Chest Stretch

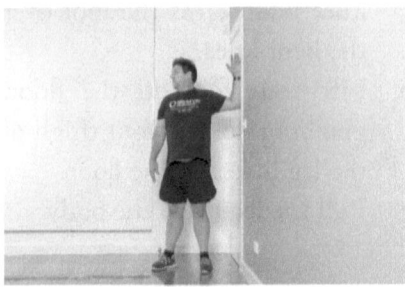

Figure 42. Chest stretch.

a. Place your arm in a bent position as show in the diagram, against a wall/pole or doorway.

b. Keep the elbow at the same height as the shoulder.

c. Rotate your body away from your arm so you feel the stretch through the chest.

d. Looking at your hand, draw a deep breath in.

e. As you rotate your head to look away from your arm, breathe out.

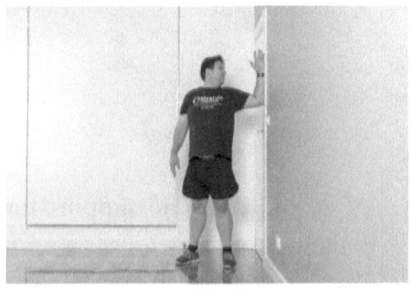

Figure 43. When doing your chest stretch, you can mobilise the neck by slowly rotating it.

a. Place your arm in a bent position, as shown in the diagram, against a wall, pole, or doorway.

b. Keep the elbow at the same height as the shoulder.

c. Rotate your body away from your arm so you feel the stretch through the chest.

d. Looking at your hand, draw a deep breath.

e. As you rotate your head to look away from your arm, breathe out.

SUPERFICIAL FRONT LINE

IT RUNS FROM the tops of the toes up to the pelvis and then connects the abdominals and thoracic cage to the neck muscles that wrap around the back of the skull. It opposes the posterior line. The main function of this sling is to curl the body up into the foetal position. When this sling becomes dysfunctional, it will cause postural problems such as forward head positioning, excessive kyphosis, and posterior pelvic tilt which, in turn, can weaken the posterior sling muscles.

This sling is the one that tends to drive poor posture. When muscles in the neck and chest regions are short and tight, they'll affect posture. Therefore it's essential to enhance a neutral spine. By doing this, you'll also strengthen the muscles in the posterior sling, reprogramming the muscles in the anterior sling to function correctly.

Stretches for Anterior Sling Muscles

Passive Chest Stretch

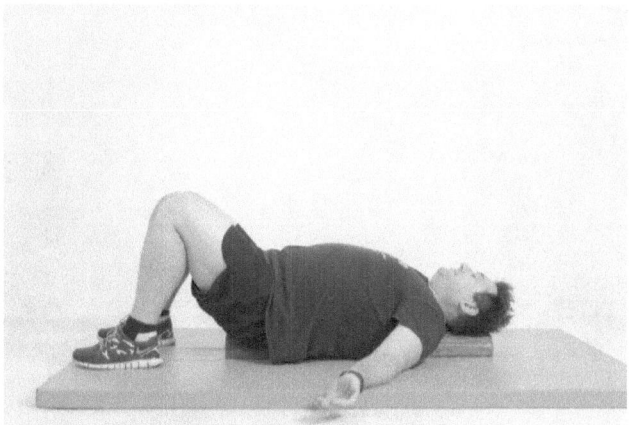

Figure 44. Lying on the roller with your arms out wide will passively stretch the chest.

a. Lie on the D-shaped foam roller lengthwise so your head and pelvis are on the roller.

b. Stretch your arms out wide so your arms and hands are on the floor.

Quad Stretch

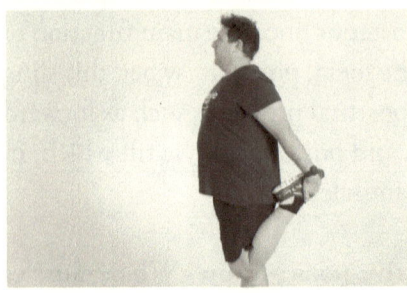 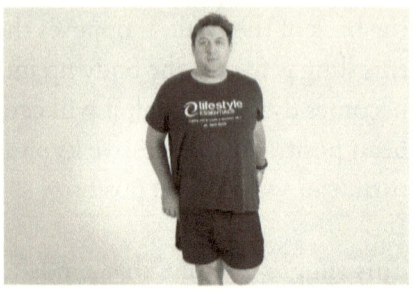

Figure 45. Quad stretch – ensure you push your hips forwards.　　*Figure 46. Quad stretch – ensure you keep your knees together.*

a. Standing up tall, hold on to a pole or wall.
b. Lift your ankle to your backside, holding on to your foot.
c. Bring your knees together.
d. Push your hips forwards, and squeeze your butt tight while pulling your foot to your backside.

Hip Flexor Stretch

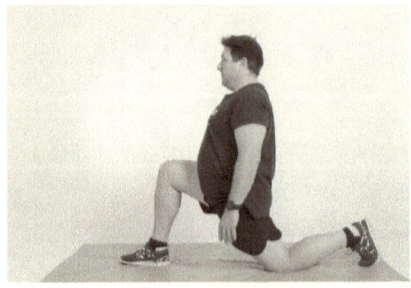 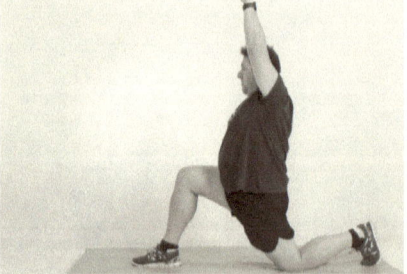

Figure 47. Hip flexor stretch.

a. Kneel on the floor with one foot in front of the other. (Ensure the foot is in front of the knee.)
b. Tuck your hips under your body, and rock your weight forwards over your front leg.

c. Once you're in position and stable, lift your arm into the air on the side of the body in which the knee is on the floor.

Chest and Neck Stretch

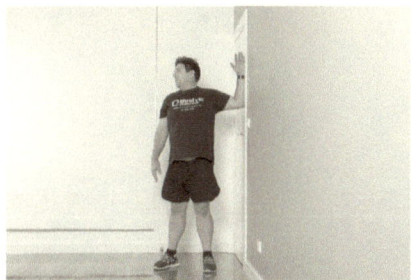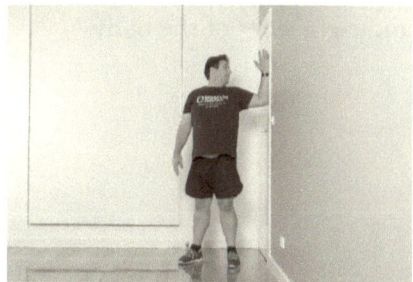

Figure 48. Chest stretch with neck mobilisation.

a. Stand up straight with your arm in a stop sign position and with your elbow at the level of the shoulder or below.
b. Rotate the body away from your arm so you're feeling a mild stretch in your chest.
c. Look at your hand, and breathe in. As you breathe out, rotate your head so you're looking away from your arm.
d. As you breathe in, look back towards your hand.

Lateral Train

The lateral sling runs down the side of your body, starting at the neck and connecting to the muscles in between the ribs to the abdominals. It then continues to the hips down the side of the leg to the foot. The major role of the oblique train is 'balance', aiding in the weight distribution between the left and right legs. It also supports the formation of the arch of the foot.

The muscles in this sling that cross the hip are essentially used for stabilisation. When muscles such as the gluteus maximus (big buttock muscle) don't work correctly, other smaller muscles need to work harder to help stabilise the hip. This can often lead to lower back pain, knee problems, and ongoing dysfunction through the lower back, hips, and knees.

Dysfunction in this sling will often lead to imbalances between the left and right sides of the body.

FUNCTIONAL SLINGS

MYERS USES THE term 'function slings' for the two muscle slings that cross over the body like an X. As mentioned, there are back and front lines. Although these slings do not play a major part in supporting posture, their actions can distort posture, such as rolling shoulders forwards. However, these slings do have an extremely important role in postural stabilisation when moving.

Front Functional Sling

The front functional sling, is for a connection between the arms and the legs through the torso. It allows movements such as throwing a ball or hitting with a bat. Although this unit is not directly related to supporting your posture, when it doesn't function correctly, it can lead to an increase in load on the deep spinal muscles. An example of this is in throwing a ball. As you throw a ball, you use this sling at the same time as the muscle around your spine that allows you to turn. If the muscles in the functional sling aren't working correctly, there's an increased workload in the deep back muscles through the rotational movement in the throwing action.

Back Functional Sling

One functional sling is across the back (posterior sling). This links your large back muscles (latissimus dorsi), the buttock muscles (gluteal muscles), and the hamstrings. Like the front sling, it is specifically involved in movements of the arm such as throwing or hitting a ball.

Although it's not directly involved in your standing posture, it does support postural muscles, attaching to the connective tissue of the lower spine and pelvic region. When this muscle train doesn't work, it means the deeper spinal muscles carry a greater load.

SPIRAL LINE

THIS MUSCLE TRAIN starts on the back of the neck, connecting the deep neck muscles to the deep shoulder muscles. This continues by wrapping around the front of the body and connecting the abdominals. Then it crosses over the body and travels down the front of the legs and wraps under the foot. It then joins the deep calf muscles connecting to the hamstrings and then travels up the spine (figure 20).

Functionally, this muscle train supports the body's movement in multiple directions, connecting the arch of the foot to the angle of the pelvis to ensure your knee is working. It sets the foundation for movements such as twisting, rotating, and side bending. When this sling isn't working properly, the body will need to compensate to carry out these movements.

Deep Front Line

This topic is extremely specialised and complex for the purpose of this book. But it's essential for you to understand that the body is a system of connections, and if one of the connections isn't working correctly, it can cause problems in other areas of the body.

If you wish to understand more about muscle trains, I would suggest you purchase *Anatomy Trains* by Thomas Myers. Although this is a textbook for a number of exercise physiology university courses, it's not too complex to read.

Breathing

It's OK to look fat while you breathe.

John came into the clinic with shoulder and lower back pain; he worked at a desk designing and wiring sound systems. John had experienced pain for over fifteen years. Over six weeks of treatment, we elevated his lower back pain. However, although the shoulder pain had reduced, it hadn't completely gone away. John did a lot of research about how to heal himself. He discovered an article on breathing and started doing correct breathing pattern exercises. Doing each of these exercises 2–3 times a day, the residual pain in his shoulder was completely gone in a period of two weeks. As much as I did help, John reduced some of this pain himself. It was his research and the application of correct breathing techniques that eliminated his pain.

In the vain world in which we live, we often try to look slimmer than we really are, either by sucking in our stomach or wearing tight clothes that hold us in, making us look thinner. There's even slimming underwear that will hold it all in for us. This pursuit of the perfect look has led to incorrect breathing patterns. So what? When we breathe the wrong way, it's only a matter of time before dysfunction will develop. There are numerous effects on the body such as a reduction in lung capacity, an increase in muscle tightness, poor posture, and an increased sensitivity to pain.

Oxygen is the basic building block of life. Breathing is the mechanism used to deliver oxygen into our body. If you don't breathe correctly, pain relief will be short-lived, and the dysfunction will not subside. This said, breathing is rarely mentioned or assessed by treating therapists. Breathing is also essential for the oxygenation of the body's cells, specifically muscles, and if they don't receive enough oxygen, they'll become dysfunctional.

The correct breathing pattern is known as diaphragmatic breathing. This is where the diaphragm draws downwards, causing a decrease in the atmospheric pressure in the lungs to be lower than the pressure outside the body.

The diaphragm functions in breathing

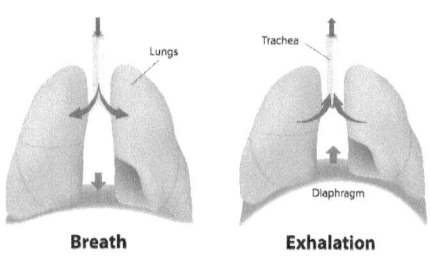

Figure 49. Correct breathing patterns are essential in preventing back pain.

This negative pressure inside the lungs causes a vacuumlike effect, drawing air into the lungs. From outside the body, you'll see a person who is diaphragmatically breathing because their stomach will rise, and then their chest will expand. The opposite occurs when breathing out. The diaphragm lifts, increasing the pressure in the lungs to a greater level than that outside the body, pushing air out. This all occurs because of a basic principle that a gas will move from a high pressure to a low pressure until an equilibrium is reached. Numerous muscles are involved in breathing including the diaphragm, the intercostal muscles, and numerous neck muscles (scalenes).

When a person's breathing pattern is incorrect, this will lead to postural imbalances in the ribcage and the neck. There are four types of breathing patterns: diaphragmatic, which is correct; clavicle; thoracic; and stomach breathing patterns. All can lead to postural dysfunction. Clavicle and thoracic breathing patterns don't engage the diaphragm, with the person being a shallow breather. Stomach breathing will often engage the diaphragm, but in some circumstances, there's no expansion of the chest, which is usually related to tight chest muscles. The diaphragmatic breathing cycle aids in the activation of the parasympathetic nervous system, which is essential in relaxing and healing muscles as well as reducing pain.

The diaphragm works closely with the pelvic floor and TVA to help support the back (the inner unit). Therefore it would make sense that if a person isn't breathing correctly (not diaphragmatically), then other muscles associated with the lower back will be affected. The diaphragm is also connected to the neck muscle via the deep frontal muscle sling. Hence dysfunction in the diaphragm will lead to these neck muscles becoming tight, leading to headaches, and a reduction in the range of movement of the neck.

The vagus nerve is one of the body's cranial nerves. It helps the body recover as well as activate the parasympathetic nervous system. When a person doesn't breathe correctly, the vagus nerve's ability to function is affected, and this can cause the incorrect activation of the pelvic muscles (psoas muscles). These muscles are involved in contributing to excessive lordosis, often associated with back pain. By breathing correctly, the vagus nerve is able to function, and postural imbalances don't happen.

Exercise in Breathing Correctly

TVA Breathing

The correct technique is termed 'diaphragmatic breathing'. As you breathe in, your stomach should push out first, and then your chest should expand. A lot of people only breathe from their chest. You can see this in more detail on our *Back Pain Eliminator* DVD series.

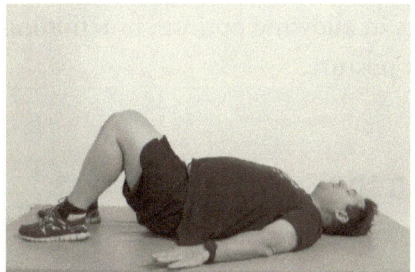 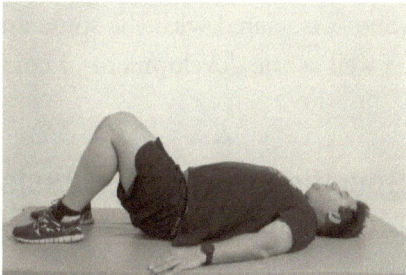

Figure 50. Diaphragmatic breathing.

MOVEMENT AND MOBILISATION

THE HUMAN BODY is designed to move, hunt, and gather, not sit behind a desk looking at a screen for hours on end. If a part of your body doesn't function properly, it's called a dysfunction. When you stop moving, dysfunction starts to develop; muscles, tendons, ligaments, and joint capsules weaken and even waste away. Joints become stiffer and lose viscosity. All of this accumulates in an inability to freely move.

Ensuring that the body can move is an essential part of the rehabilitation process associated with any back pain condition. Mobilising joints helps increase blood flow and the supply of extra nutrients to the area while preventing joint stiffness and joint locking. Mobilising the spine and the joints associated with the spine assists in allowing optimal functioning as well as the development of correct posture.

Specific Exercises to Assist in the Mobilisation of the Spine

Vertical Foam Roller

This exercise is a great way to mobilise the lumbar spine and the sacroiliac joint. It works as though you were wringing out a towel, rotating the spine from the top down and the bottom up at the same time. When doing this exercise, all movements should be small and controlled so you don't fall off the roller. The exercise can be beneficial if you have a budge or a prolapse, but the movements *must* be small and slow.

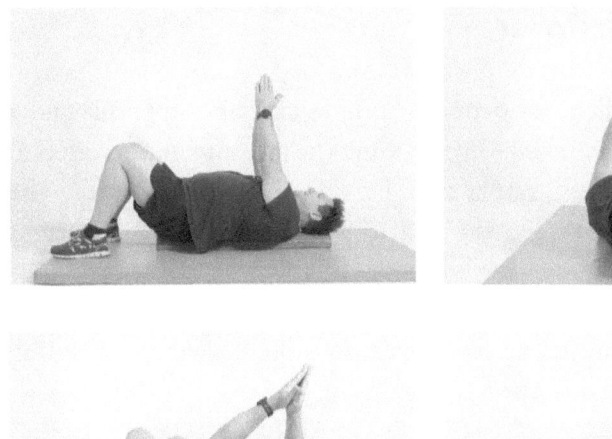
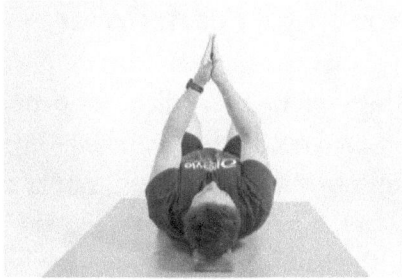
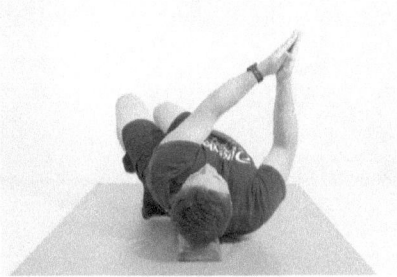
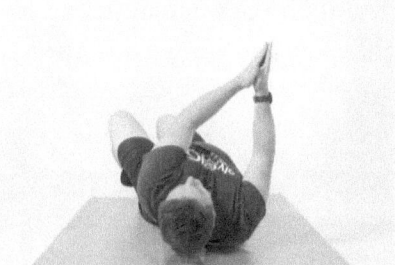

Figure 51. The vertical foam roller is a great way to mobilise the spine.

1. Lie on the D-shaped foam roller lengthwise so your head and the base of your spine are both on the roller.
2. Place your arms in the air, palms together, and your feel flat on the floor, hips wide apart.
3. Gently rock your arms from one side to the other. As you rock, allow your knees to travel in the opposite direction to the arms.
4. Start with small movements, and slowly increase the range of movement as the spine's mobility increases.
5. Ensure you breathe slowly and rhythmically with the movements.

Horizontal Foam Roller

This exercise is excellent for people who have excessive kyphosis and a forward head carriage. It helps by reloading the pressure in the vertebral discs so they're balanced, rather than locking the spine forwards. The essential part of this exercise is to start just below your armpit height at the base of the scapula. As you move the roller up the spine, move in small increments so it mobilises each of the spine's vertebral joints. Travel up the spine until you feel there's no more benefit to extending the spine and the head is just moving.

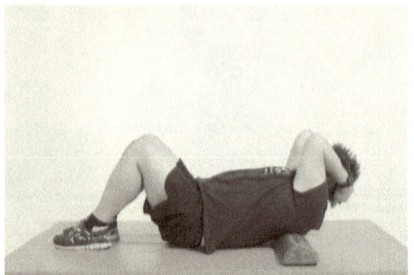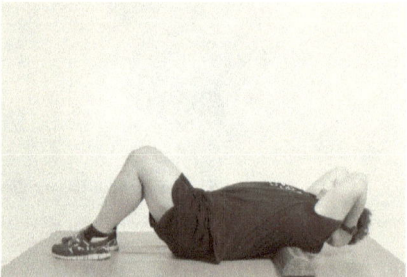

Figure 52. Thoracic mobilisation.

1. Lie on your back with your knees bent. Place the D-shaped foam roller across your back at the height of the bottom of the shoulder blade (scapula).
2. Place your hands behind your head, with your elbows pointing up towards the ceiling.
3. As you breathe out, relax backwards (arching your back), only moving as far back as you can without any pain.
4. As you breathe in, draw yourself up.
5. Repeat three or four times, and then rest so the roller moves up your spine towards your head. As you move up the spine, it's like moving up only one segment of the vertebra at a time.
6. Repeat the movements in steps 3 and 4 at each level of the vertebrae.

Thoracic Mobilisation

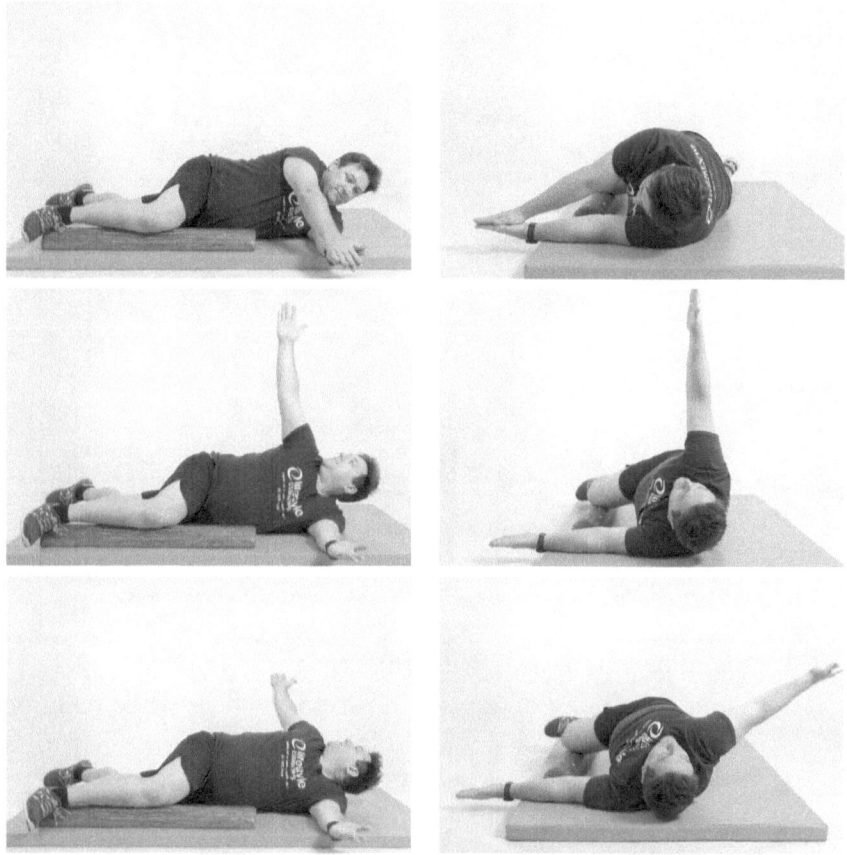

Figure 53. Thoracic mobilisation.

1. Lie on your side with your top leg bent at ninety degrees at the hip.
2. Place both arms out in front of you as shown in the first diagram.
3. Keeping your knee in contact with the roller and your bottom arm on the floor, slowly sweep your top arm across your body.
4. Keep your nose in line with the moving arm.
5. Sweep your top arm over your body as far as you can travel without lifting your other knee off the roller.

The Lewitt Technique

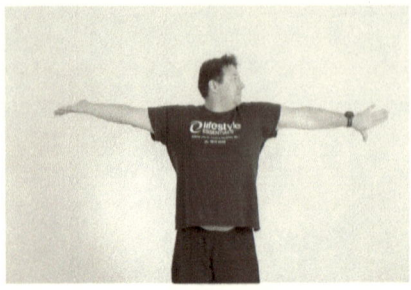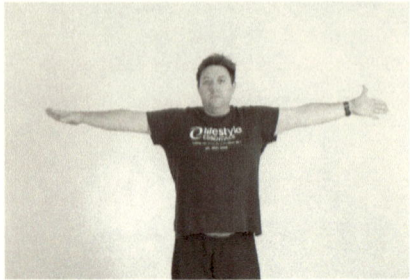

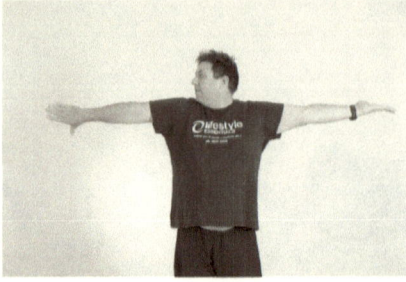

Figure 54. The Lewitt technique aids in the mobilisation of the neck muscles.

1. Stand or sit tall, with your arms straight to the side.
2. Point the thumb of one arm down to the floor while pointing up the other arm's palm towards the ceiling.
3. Look at the hand with the thumb pointing down.
4. Inhale deeply. As you breathe out, rotate your head from one side to the other, and simultaneously rotate your hands into the opposite position (thumb down turns to palm up, and the other moves from palm up to thumb down).
5. Breathe in and then rotate your head from side to side, simultaneously rotating your hands into the opposite position.

ELIMINATING BACK PAIN

THERE ARE TWO essential elements to understand about back pain:

1. If you have a structural problem in your spine, it's unlikely that you can eliminate it without surgery. However, this doesn't mean you can't live pain-free. With the right treatment and exercises, anyone can live their life pain-free.
2. Simply reading this book will *not* reduce or eliminate your back pain; you need to apply the principles in the book, or they just won't work.

So the question you must ask yourself is this – are you prepared to take the journey and do the things necessary to reduce and eliminate your back pain? This is a 'yes or no' question, no ifs, ands, or buts. Otherwise, it just won't work. You must be committed to take action using the information in this program.

So we need you to set a back pain elimination *goal*. Yes, a goal! Let's set what is called a 'WASPIER goal'.

The *W*: Why. Why are you setting this goal? What is your why? To be pain-free is a good why, but it's not motivational enough. Think of what being pain-free means to you, your life, and your family.

What are your three whys (reasons) for being pain-free?

The *A*: Accountable. Who are you accountable to? It can be a personal trainer, a therapist, a family member, or one of our back pain consultants. It doesn't matter who, but *you need to be accountable to somebody*. Tell this person your goal and how you need to be kept accountable.

Who can *you* be accountable to?

The *S*: **SMART Goal.** Set a SMART goal, and have a *s*pecific outcome. For example, decrease pain from a 9 to a 4 in four weeks. Make the goal *m*easureable so you know where you're at and whether you're making progress or regressing. It's essential to make your goal *a*chievable and *r*ealistic. Your goal may be just to do your exercises every day (and not focus on pain). This is a great goal as you're in control of your actions in this way, more so than your pain levels. Finally, it must be *t*imed. Choose a specific date to work towards, for example, 1 July 2017.

What is your SMART goal?

The *P*: **Present Tense.** Achieving a goal is about believing you can, so the *P* stands for living in the present moment as if you have already achieved your goal. This means no more declaring you have back pain, no more living your life through the eyes of your pain. Yes, you need to respect where you're at. But every morning get up with the 'I don't have back pain and never will' attitude.

The *I*: **Inspiration.** Does your goal inspire you? As a back pain elimination goal, you may make little goals to get you started, such as doing your exercises every day. But if the thought of achieving your goal doesn't inspire you, then you need to get a better goal. I'm sure the thought of being able to lift your baby without pain or to sleep all night is inspirational enough to motivate you to do what it takes. If not, get a bigger goal.

Does the thought of achieving this SMART goal inspire you to do what it takes?

The *E*: **Effect.** What effect will achieving this goal have on your life? Make a list of what your life would look like if you achieved this goal. Then make a list of the effects on your life that may occur if you *don't* achieve this goal. Then compare both lists.

The *R*: **Record.** You should keep track of your progress and your results weekly so you can trace the changes that have occurred.

Use a notebook and record your actions and progress daily as a guide to help you achieve your goals.

Now that we have a goal, let's set up an action plan to eliminate your pain.

Step 1. Turn off the pain

As discussed earlier, the way to control pain is via the parasympathetic nervous system. Being active increases the PNS and reduces the SNS, so you'll be able to desensitise your pain response.

- Reduce stress.
- Breathe correctly (slow diaphragmatic breathing).
- Do meditation walking. Breathe in for a number of steps, and then breathe out for the same number of steps. Then breathe in for four steps and out for another four.
- Do exercises that are specifically parasympathetically dominant.

The exercises below, in my opinion, are the best parasympathetic exercises.

TVA Breathing

This can be done on a foam roller or on the floor.

1. Lie on your back with your knees bent.
2. Push out your stomach as though it's bloated.
3. Take a deep breath.
4. As you breathe out, draw your stomach in.
5. Push out your stomach as you breathe in; draw your stomach in as you breathe out.

Four- Point Stand

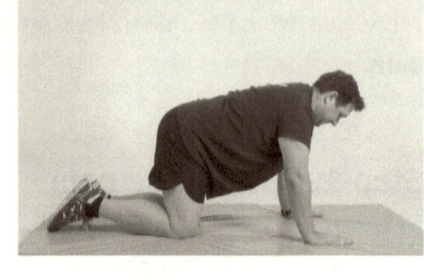

1. Activate your TVA by drawing in your abdomen.
2. Take the weight out of the opposite arm and leg, but keep the hand and knee in contact with the floor.
3. Alternate from one side to the other, taking the weight out of the opposite arm and leg.
4. Try not to let the hips rotate or move. Keep them straight and still.

Click or scan the link below to view a video on how to do the decompression four-point stance

https://www.stopbackpain.com.au/stop-back-pain-four-point-stance

Leg Extension Neural Mobilisation

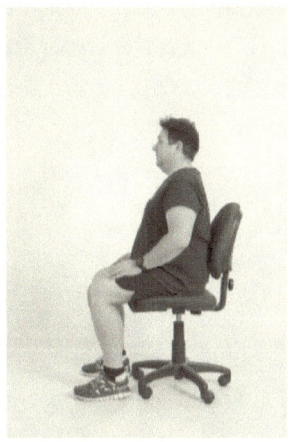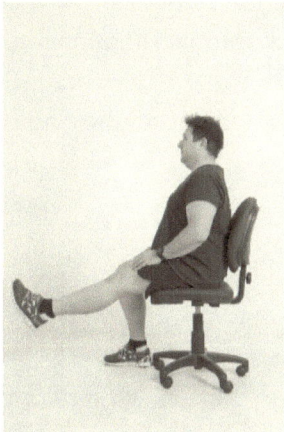

1. Sit up straight on a chair (like a piece a string is drawing you up the ceiling) with your feet flat on the floor.
2. Still sitting upright, slowly extend your leg. (Make sure this is slow and only as far as you can go that does not cause pain in your back; pulling is OK.)
3. Return the foot to the floor.

Step 2. Develop a neutral spine

Developing a neutral spine is a long-term program. You can't change your posture in the short term. You need to continually work on improving your posture. To learn about developing a neutral spine, we'll look at various programs for different types of posture. There are number of different postures to consider.

1. Excessive kyphosis is when there's an overcurvature of the upper back (thoracic region).
2. Excessive lordosis is when there's an overcurvature of the lower back (lumbar region).
3. Flat back is when there's a lack of curvature in the spine.

When a muscle isn't functioning at its optimal level, the best approach is to isolate the muscle to work independently and then integrate that muscle back into its functional unit. This way, the structure will work correctly. This is how we approach any exercise program that is related to rehabilitation and improving posture.

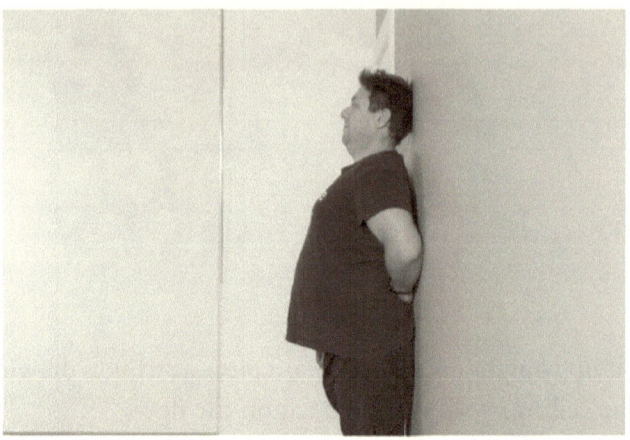

Figure 55. Wall stance is a good way to assess your postural curves.

1. Stand with your heel, hips, shoulders, and head against the wall as shown above. Your posture may not allow you to do this. If so, focus on either the lower or upper part of the spine.
2. Place your hand behind your back in the region of the natural curve of your spine.
3. Ideally, for a correct neutral spine, you'll only be able to slide your hand behind your back to your knuckles.

If you can slide your hand in further, there's too much curve (lordosis).

1. Place your hand behind your back until your knuckles are under your vertebrae.
2. Imagine you have headlights on your backside. Turn them down towards your heels, and this will reduce the excessive curve in the spine. Hold your pelvis in this position for 30–45 seconds, and repeat 4–5 times throughout the day.

If you can't slide your hand under your back, it's flat, without a curve.

1. Imagine you have headlights on your backside; turn the headlights up towards your head, and this will increase the curve in the spine.
2. Place your hand behind your back so your knuckles are under your vertebrae.
3. Hold your pelvis in this position for 30–45 seconds, and repeat 4–5 times throughout the day.

Correct Exercises for Excessive Kyphosis

Mobilisation and activation exercises that can help reduce excessive kyphosis are as follows.

Vertical Foam Roller

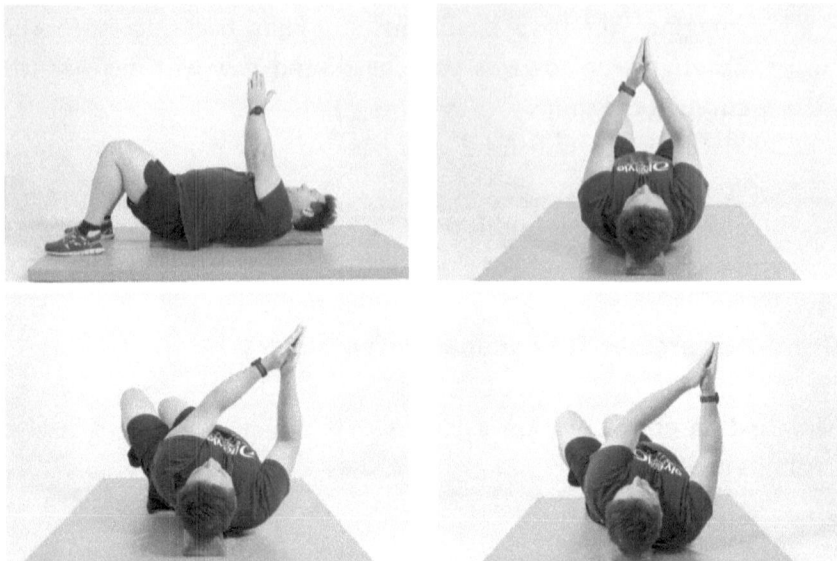

Figure 56. The vertical foam roller is a great way to mobilise the spine.

1. Lie on the D-shaped foam roller lengthwise so your head and the base of your spine are both on the roller.
2. Place your arms in the air, palms together, and your feel flat on the floor, hips wide apart.
3. Gently rock your arms from one side to the other. As you rock, allow your knees to travel in the opposite direction to the arms.
4. Start with small movements, and slowly increase the range of movement as the spine's mobility increases.
5. Ensure you breathe slowly and rhythmically with the movements.

Horizontal Foam Roller

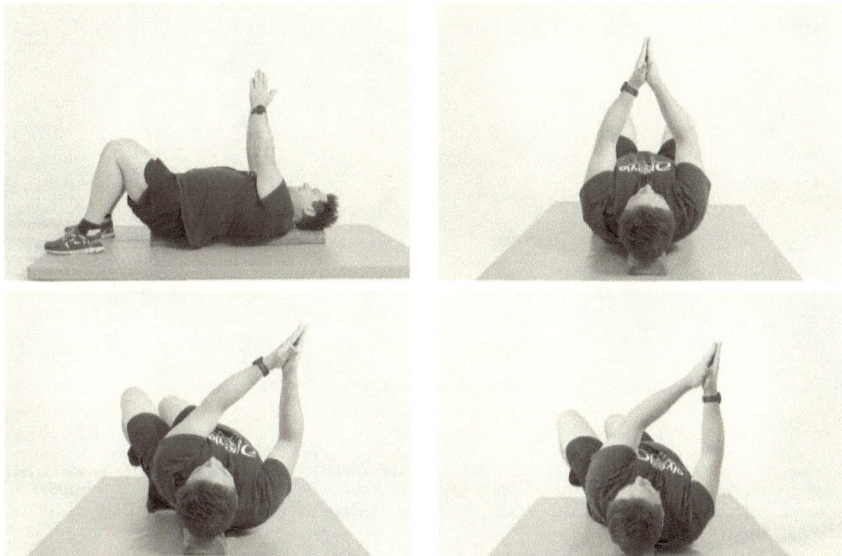

Figure 57. The vertical foam roller is a great way to mobilise the spine.

1. Lie on your back with your knees bent. Place the D-shaped foam roller across your back at the height of the bottom of the shoulder blade (scapula).
2. Place your hands behind your head, with your elbows pointing up towards the ceiling.
3. As you breathe out, relax backwards (arching your back), only moving as far back as you can without any pain.
4. As you breathe in, draw yourself up.
5. Repeat three or four times, and then rest so the roller moves up your spine towards your head. As you move up the spine, it's like moving up only one segment of the vertebra at a time.
6. Repeat the movements in steps 3 and 4 at each level of the vertebrae.

McKenzie Press

Don't do this exercise if you have any disc injuries.

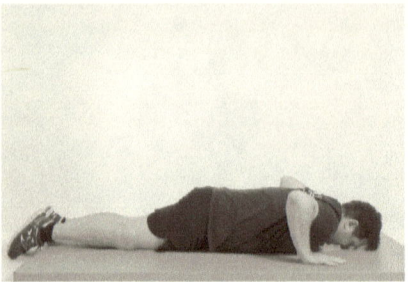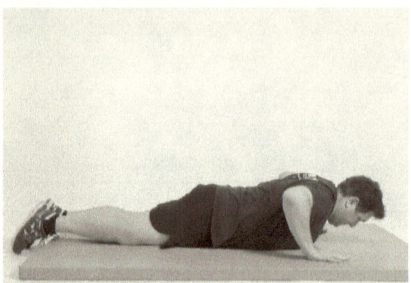

Figure 58. The McKenzie press helps reduce the thoracic spine.

1. Lie on your stomach with your hands in the push-up position.
2. Push up through your arms so you take the weight out of your chest. (Note: you're not lifting from your lower back.)
3. Pull your shoulder blades back and together, hold yourself up, and take your weight out of your hands. (Weight is transferred into the upper back, not the lower back.)
4. Keep your chin tucked in the whole time so you're looking down.
5. Hold for thirty seconds to start with, and repeat 2–4 times throughout the day.

Foetal Reflex Prone Cobra

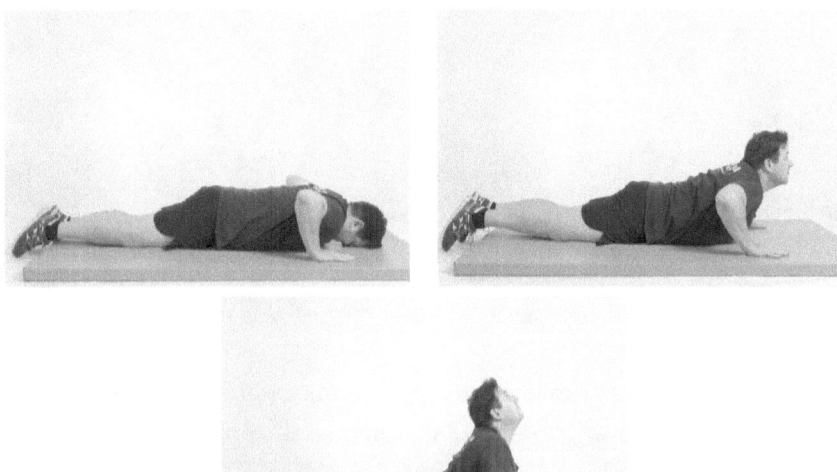

Figure 59. This exercise uses the foetal reflex to extend your upper back.

1. Lie on your stomach.
2. Roll your head up so your eyes travel across the floor and up the wall to the ceiling.
3. Once your head gets to its full range of movement, push up through your arms into the cobra position.
4. Travel up as high as you can while being pain-free.
5. When rolling down, return the chest to the floor first, and then return the head to the neutral position.

Superman Posterior Sling

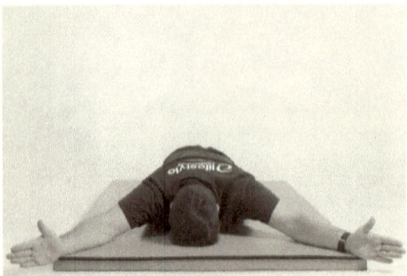 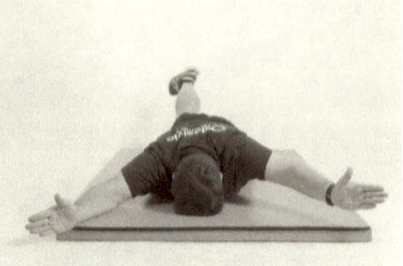

Figure 60. Superman, strengthening and activating the posterior.

1. Lie on your stomach with your arms extended out on a forty-five-degree angle at the shoulder, pointing your thumbs up towards the ceiling.
2. Squeeze your glutes (butt); lift your opposite arm and leg off the floor (2–3 cm off the floor) with your thumb pointing up.
3. Return to the floor.
4. Alternate sides.

NEURAL MOBILISATION

Chest-Neck Mobilisation (Lewitt Technique)

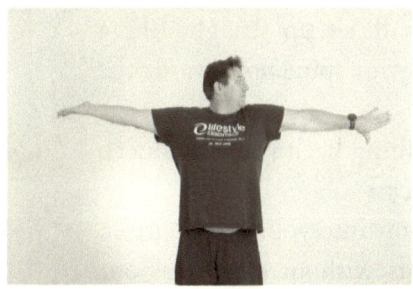 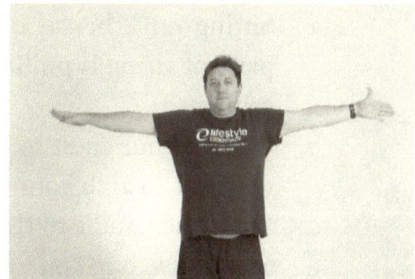

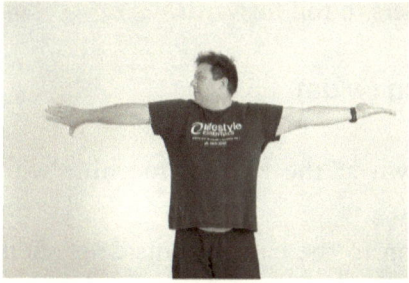

Figure 61. Lewitt technique, mobilisation of the neck.

1. Stand or sit tall, with your arms straight to the side.
2. Point down the thumb of one arm to the floor while pointing up the other arm's palm towards the ceiling.
3. Look at the hand with the thumb pointing down.
4. Inhale deeply. As you breathe out, rotate your head from one side to the other, and simultaneously rotate your hands into the opposite position (thumb down turns to palm up, and the other moves from palm up to thumb down).
5. Breathe in and then rotate your head from side to side, simultaneously rotating your hands into the opposite position.

Strength Exercises that Can Help
Reduce Excessive Kyphosis

1. **Seated row**

    a. Sitting on a bench or ball, sit up straight like a piece of string is pulling your spine up towards the ceiling.
    b. Puff up your chest by pulling back your shoulders. (Try not to arch your back.)
    c. Draw the handle of the row into your belly button.
    d. Straighten out your arms without allowing your shoulders to roll forwards.

2. **Lat pull down (wide)**

    a. Sit down at the lat pull machine with the wide grip bar.
    b. Grab on to the bar just outside of shoulder width apart.
    c. Draw your elbows down towards the floor so your arms are next to your body.
    d. Extend your arms so they're straight (without lifting your shoulders).

3. **Reverse flies (band)**

    a. Standing up tall, like a piece of string is pulling your spine up towards the ceiling.
    b. Holding your arms out in front and pull the weight outwards like you're opening up your arms for a hug (pull the arms out the side of your body.
    c. Try not to let your head move forwards.
    d. Slowly return your arms to the starting position.

4. External rotator cuff

a. Stand up tall, like a piece of string is pulling your spine up towards the ceiling.

b. Place a towel between your elbow and stomach, with your elbow bent at ninety degrees.

c. Pull your hand out sideways from the body, keeping the elbow against the body.

d. Try not to drop the towel, and ensure you keep the elbow bent.

e. Return the hand back to the starting position across your body.

Stretches that Can Help Reduce Excessive Kyphosis

1. Pectoralis major chest stretch

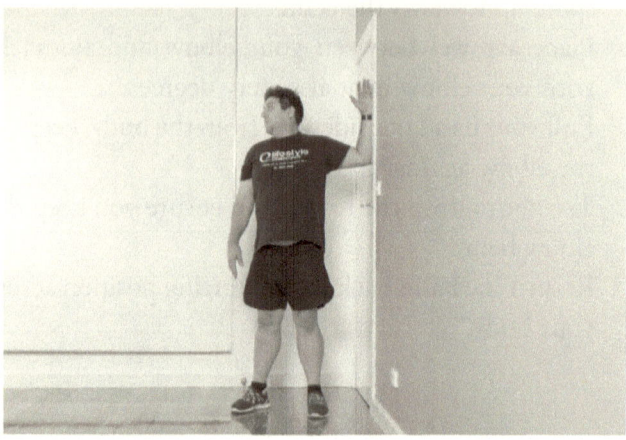

    a. Place your arm in a bent position, as shown in the diagram, against a wall, pole, or doorway.

    b. Keep the elbow at the same height as the shoulder.

    c. Looking in the opposite direction, rotate your body away from your arm so you feel the stretch through the chest.

2. Pectoralis minor chest stretch

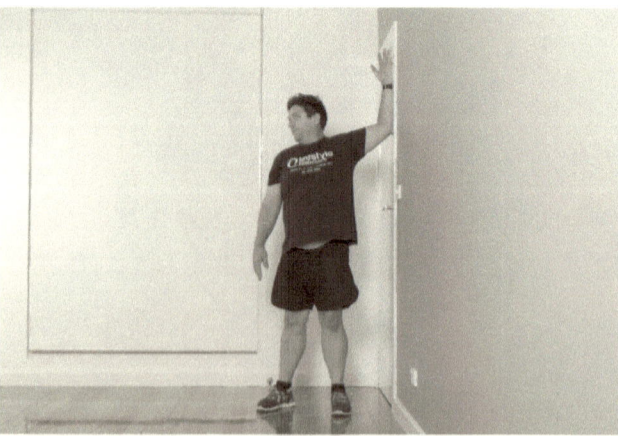

    a. Place your arm in a bent position, as shown in the diagram, against a wall, pole, or doorway.

b. Place the elbow above the height of the shoulder.
c. Looking in the opposite direction, rotate your body away from your arm so you feel the stretch through the chest.

3. Lat stretch

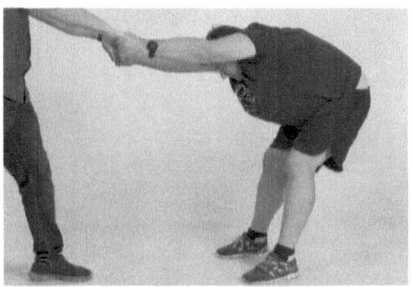 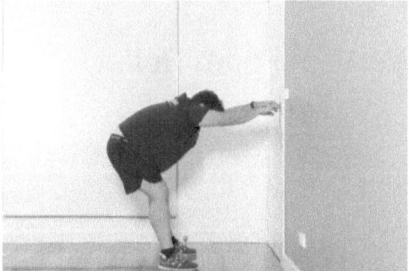

a. Hold on to a stable, solid object that can't move.
b. Sit back; taking the weight through your arms, bend your knees and bow forwards, looking down towards the floor.
c. Holding on to the object, adjust your weight to one side of the body to stretch that side.
d. Change sides.

Suggested Weekly Plan

	Mon.	Tue.	Wed.	Thur.	Fri.	Sat.
Mob.		Yes		Yes		Yes
Strength	Yes		Yes		Yes	
Stretches	Yes		Yes		Yes	

EXCESSIVE LORDOSIS

Mobilisation and activation exercises that can help reduce excessive kyphosis are as follows.

Vertical Foam Roller

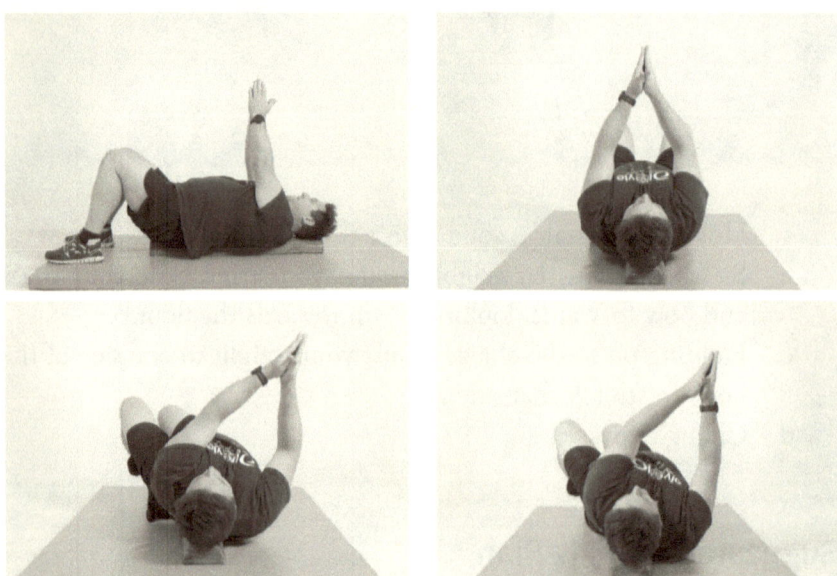

Figure 51. Vertical foam roller is a great way to mobilise the spine

1. Lie on the D-shaped foam roller lengthwise so your head and the base of your spine are both on the roller.
2. Place your arms in the air, palms together, and your feel flat on the floor, hips wide apart.
3. Gently rock your arms from one side to the other. As you rock, allow your knees to travel in the opposite direction to the arms.
4. Start with small movements, and slowly increase the range of movement as the spine's mobility increases.
5. Ensure you breathe slowly and rhythmically with the movements.

Thoracic Mobilisation

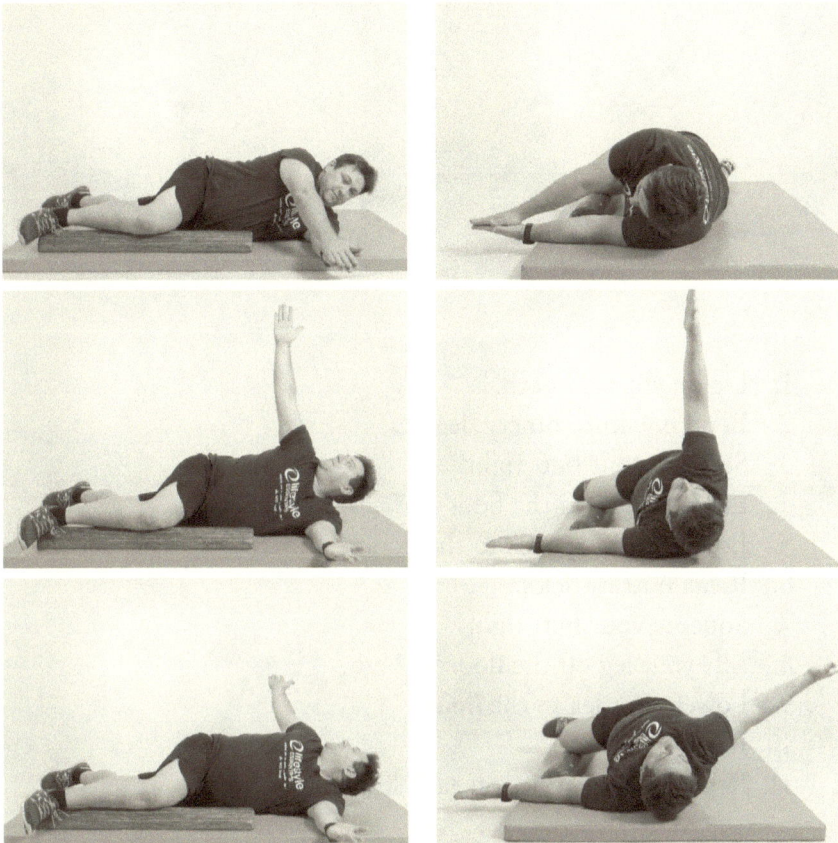

1. Lie on your side with your top leg bent at ninety degrees at the hip.
2. Place both arms out in front of you as shown in the first diagram.
3. Keeping your knee in contact with the roller and your bottom arm on the floor, slowly sweep your top arm across your body.
4. Keep your nose in line with the moving arm.
5. Sweep your top arm over your body as far as you can without lifting your other knee off the roller.

Gluteal Activation

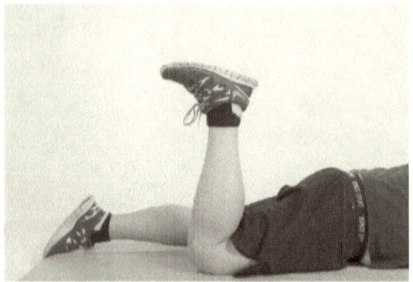 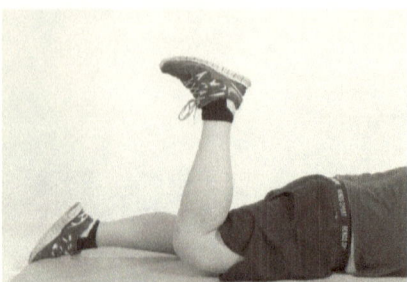

1. Lie on your stomach.
2. Bend one knee ninety degrees.
3. Squeeze your butt tight.
4. Lift your leg off the floor 2–3 cm.
5. Lower your leg back to the floor.
6. Relax butt muscles.
7. Squeeze your butt tight.
8. Lift your leg off the floor 2–3 cm.
9. Lower your leg to the floor.
10. Relax your butt.
11. Repeat 10–12 times on each leg.

TVA Activation Breathing

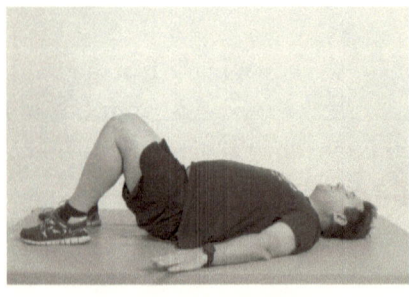 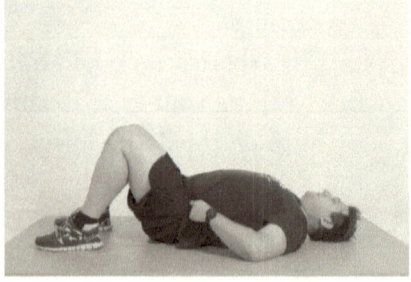

1. Lie on your back with your knees bent.
2. Push out your stomach as though it's bloated.

3. Take a deep breath.
4. As you breathe out, draw your stomach in.
5. Push out your stomach as you breathe in, and draw your stomach in as you breathe out.

Neural Mobilisation

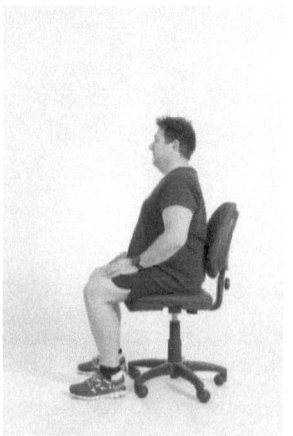 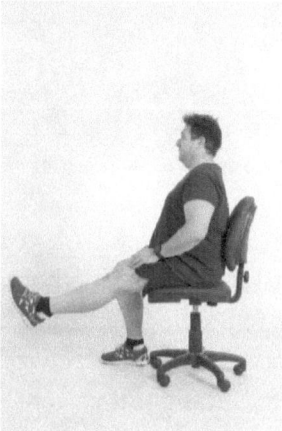

1. Sit up straight on a chair (like a piece of string is drawing you up to the ceiling) with your feet flat on the floor.
2. Keep sitting upright, and slowly extend your leg. (Make sure this is slow and only as far as you can go without causing back pain. Pulling is OK.)
3. Return the foot to the floor.

STRENGTHENING PROGRAM

1. Hip extensions

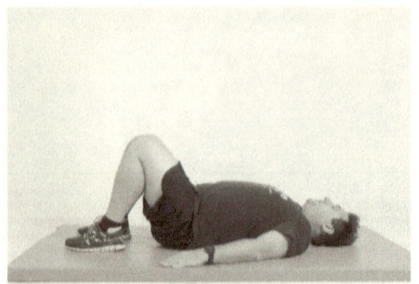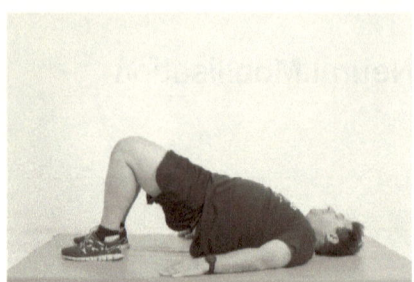

a. Lie on your back with your knees bent, feet flat on the floor.
b. Activate your pelvic floor, and squeeze your butt muscles like you're holding on to a $100 bill.
c. Once everything is activated, lift your hips off the floor. (Ideally, form a straight line from the shoulders to the knees; but if you can't go this high, start at your own level.)
d. Return to the floor and relax, and then repeat from step 2.

2. Squats

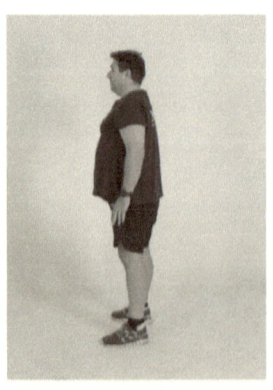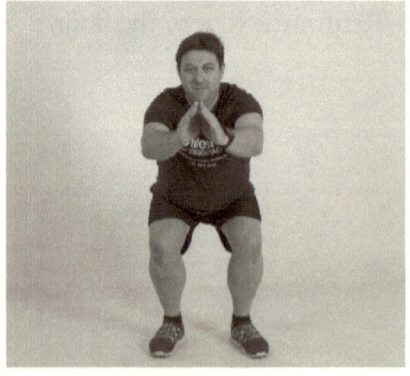

a. Stand in front of a bench or a chair, with your feet hip-width apart.
b. Sit on the bench, and then stand up.

c. Sit on the bench slowly so you touch it without actually sitting on it, and then stand up.

d. Now sit down so you touch it, but put no weight on the bench.

3. TVA heel taps

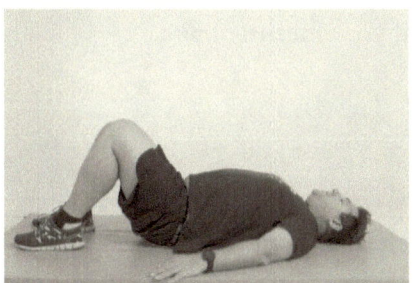 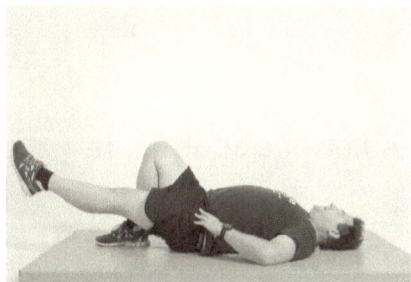

a. Lie on the floor on your back with your knees bent.

b. Turn on your pelvic floor by drawing it up as if preventing yourself from going to the bathroom. (Keep the pelvic floor turned on the whole time.)

c. Lift one leg off the floor and extend it so it's straight, and then tap your heel on the floor.

d. Return your foot to the starting position, and then repeat for the other leg.

4. TVA leg lifts

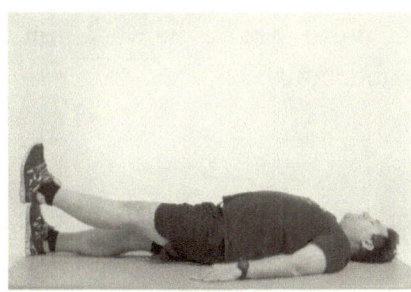 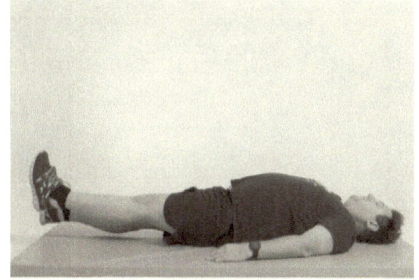

a. Lie on the floor on your back with your knees bent.

b. Turn on your pelvic floor by drawing it up as if preventing yourself from going to the bathroom. (Keep the pelvic floor turned on the whole time.)

c. Slowly lift one foot 2–3 cm. off the floor. As you put it back on the floor, lift the other foot off the floor (just before the first one touches the floor).

d. Make sure you don't arch your back as you change feet. If you need to do so, alternate feet if you're feeling pain.

5. Lower abdominals

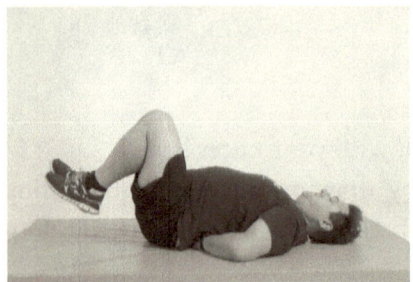 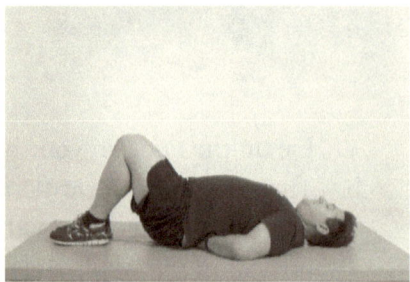

a. Lie on your back with your knees bent and your feet close to your hips.

b. Place your hand in the curve of your lower back.

c. Flatten out your back so you're pressing your spine down on your hand.

d. Keeping the pressure on your hand, lift one foot off the floor, put it back on the floor, and then alternate sides.

e. Try to keep the same pressure on your hand the whole time. (You'll feel this in your lower abdominals.)

6. Wall stance

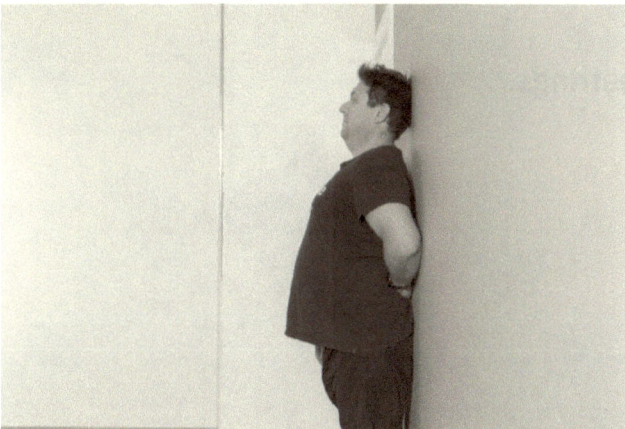

a. Stand with your heel, hips, shoulders, and head against the wall as shown above. Your posture may not allow you to do this. If so, focus on either the lower part or the upper part of the spine.
b. Place your hand behind your back until your knuckles are under your vertebrae.
c. Imagine you have headlights on your backside. Turn them down towards your heels. This will reduce the excessive curve in the spine. Hold your pelvis in this position for 30–45 seconds, and repeat 4–5 times throughout the day.

STRETCHES

1. Hamstrings

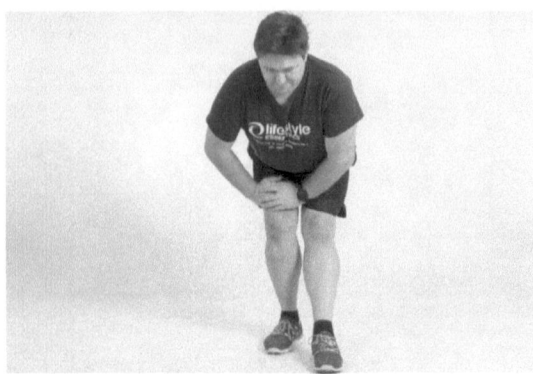

a. Place your foot in front of the other
b. Push your hips back, bending your knee at the back, keeping the front leg straight.
c. Bow forwards, tilting your hips up towards the ceiling. (You should feel a stretch in the hamstring.)

2. Glutes

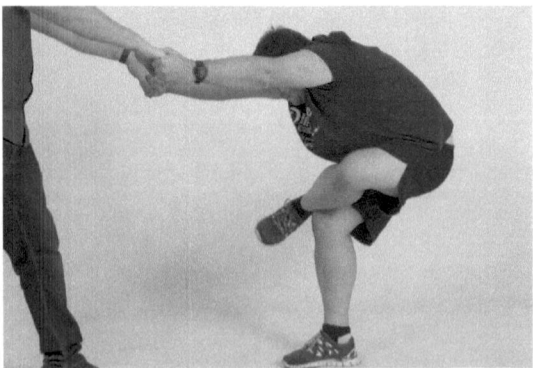

a. Hold on to a solid support for balance.
b. Cross your leg so your foot is on your opposite knee.
c. Leaning back, bend your knee as you allow yourself to sink backwards. You should feel the stretch in your backside.

3. Calf

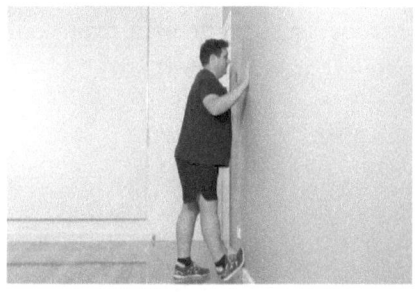 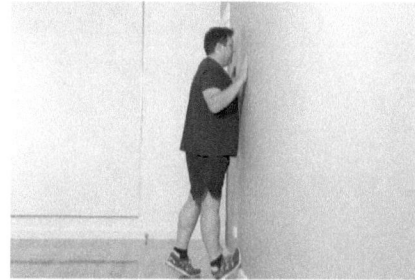

   a.   Standing up tall, place your foot against a wall or solid surface, with your toes up towards the ceiling.

   b.   Push your hips into the wall/pole.

   c.   Try not to let your heel slip backwards. You should feel a stretch in the calf.

4. Hip flexor

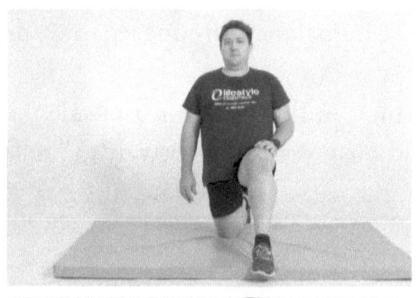 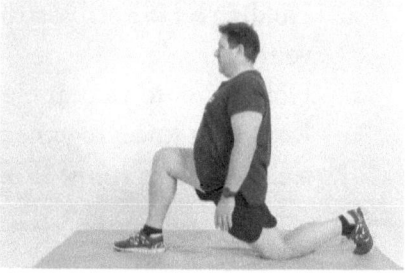

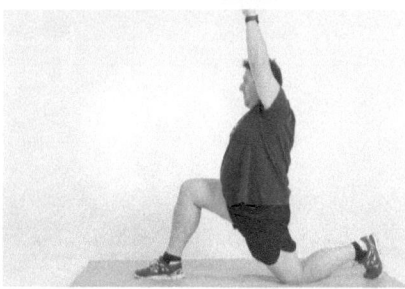 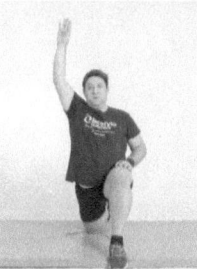

   a.   Kneel on the floor with one foot forward. (Make sure the foot is in front of the knee.)

b. Rock your weight forwards while keeping your hips tucked under your body.

c. Once your weight is over the front leg, lift the arm over your head (the opposite arm to the one that is forward).

5. Quads

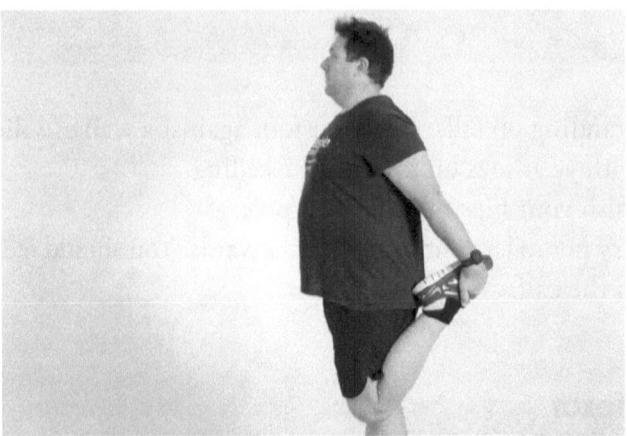

a. Holding on to a stable structure for balance, lift one leg towards your backside.

b. Holding on to your ankle or foot, pull up to your backside.

c. Keep your knees together, and push your hips forwards. You'll feel the stretch in the front of the leg.

FLAT BACK

MOBILISATION AND ACTIVATION exercises that can help reduce excessive kyphosis are as follows:

1. Vertical foam roller

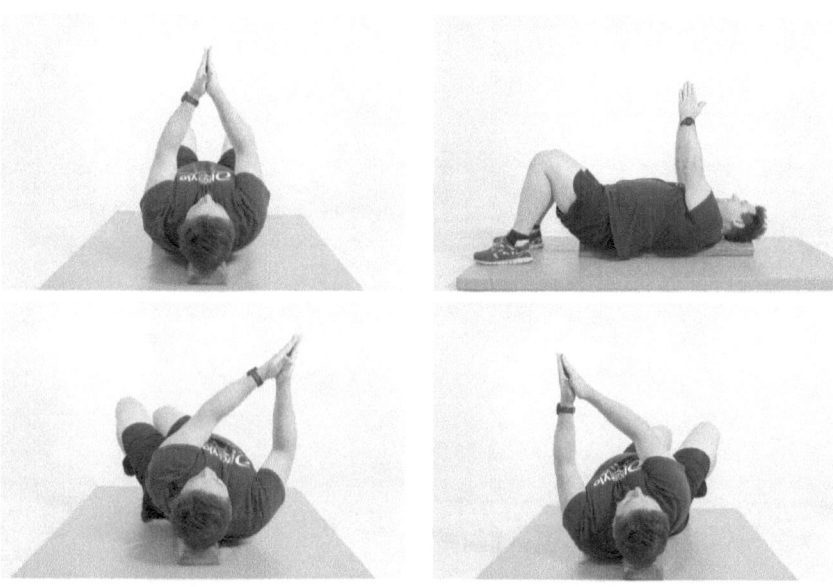

a. Lie on the D-shaped foam roller lengthwise so your head and the base of your spine are both on the roller.

b. Place your arms in the air, palms together, and your feel flat on the floor, hips wide apart.

c. Gently rock your arms from one side to the other. As you rock, allow your knees to travel in the opposite direction to the arms.

d. Start with small movements, and slowly increase the range of movement as the spine's mobility increases.

e. Ensure you breathe slowly and rhythmically with the movements.

2. Thoracic mobilisation

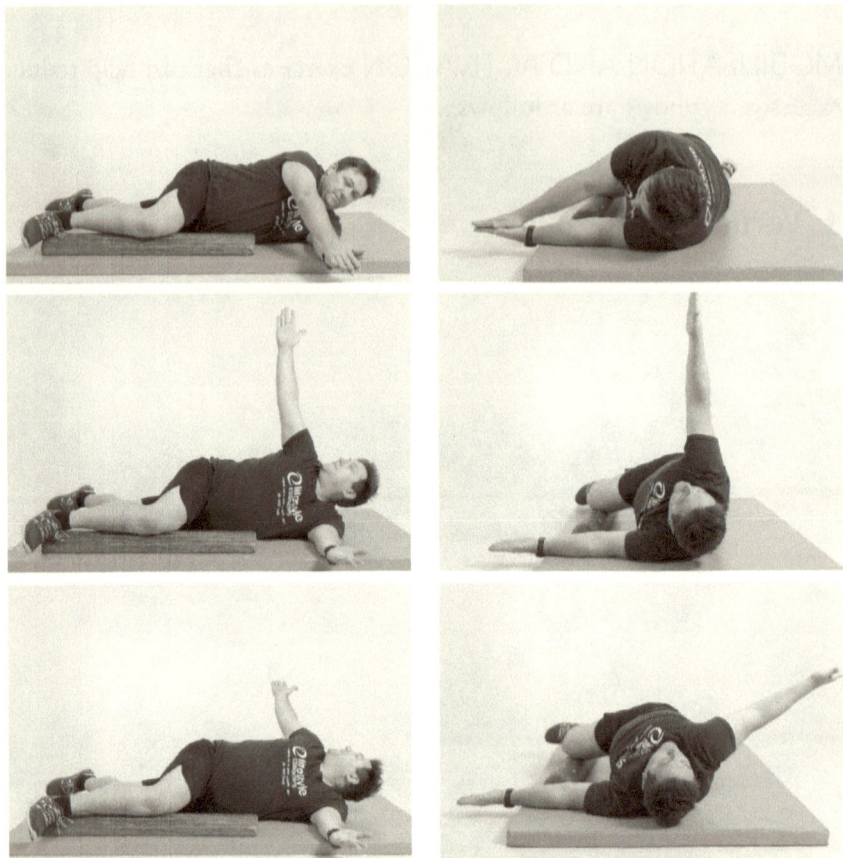

a. Lie on your side with your top leg bent at ninety degrees at the hip.

b. Place both arms out in front of you as shown in the first diagram.

c. Keeping your knee in contact with the roller and your bottom arm on the floor, slowly sweep your top arm across your body.

d. Keep your nose in line with the moving arm.

e. Sweep your top arm over your body as far as you can without lifting your other knee off the roller.

3. Gluteal activation

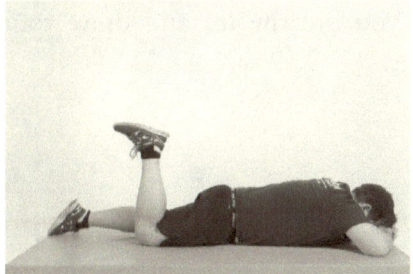
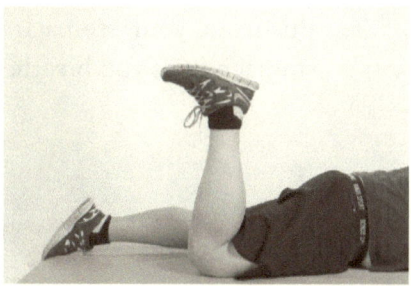
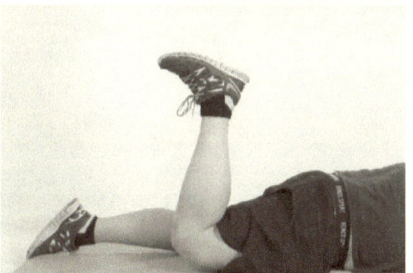

a. Lie on your stomach.
b. Bend one knee ninety degrees.
c. Squeeze your butt tight.
d. Lift your leg off the floor 2–3 cm.
e. Lower your leg back to the floor.
f. Relax your butt muscles.
g. Squeeze your butt tight.
h. Lift your leg off the floor 2–3 cm.
i. Lower your leg to the floor.
j. Relax your butt.
k. Repeat 10–12 times on each leg.

4. TVA activation breathing

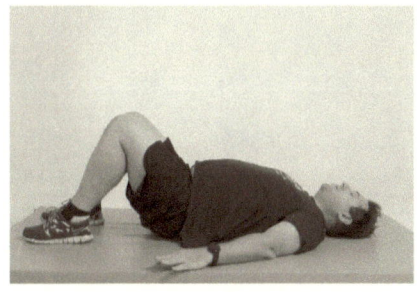
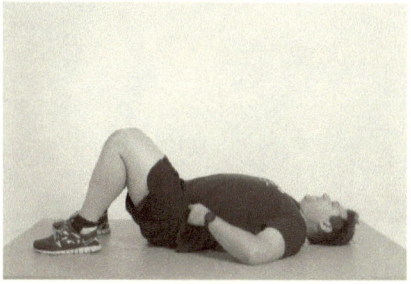

a. Lie on your back with your knees bent.
b. Push out your stomach as though it's bloated.

   c. Take a deep breath.

   d. As you breathe out, draw your stomach in.

   e. Push out your stomach as you breathe in, and draw your stomach in as you breathe out.

STRENGTHENING PROGRAM

1. Hip extensions

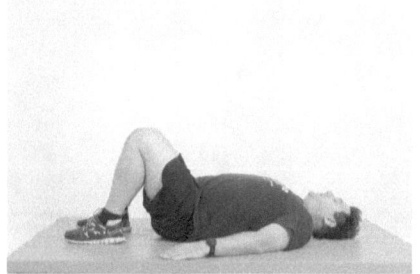 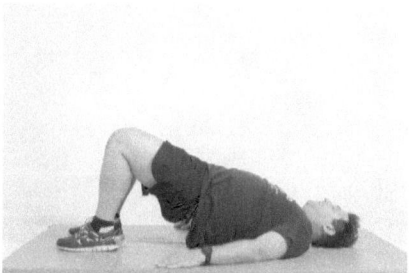

  a. Lie on your back with your knees bent, feet flat on the floor.
  b. Activate your pelvic floor, and squeeze your butt muscles like you're holding on to a $100 bill.
  c. Once everything is activated, lift your hips off the floor. (Ideally, form a straight line from the shoulders to the knees; but if you can't go this high, start at your own level.)
  d. Return to the floor and relax, and then repeat from step 2.

2. Squats

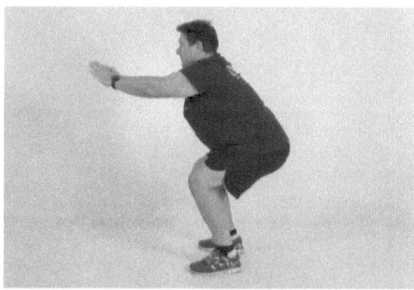

  a. Stand in front of a bench or a chair, with your feet hip width apart.
  b. Sit on the bench, and then stand up.
  c. Sit on the bench slowly so you touch it without actually sitting on it, and then stand up.

    d.   Now sit down so you touch it, but put no weight on the bench.

3. TVA heel taps

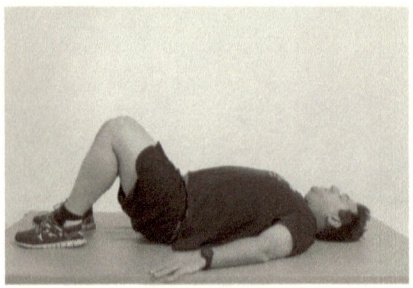 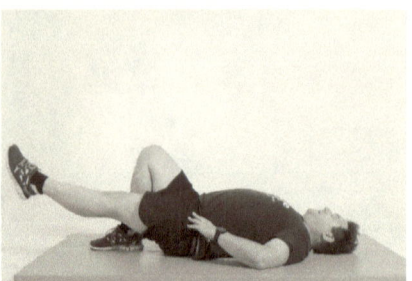

    a.   Lie on the floor on your back with your knees bent.

    b.   Turn on your pelvic floor by drawing it up as if preventing yourself from going to the bathroom. (Keep the pelvic floor turned on the whole time.)

    c.   Lift one leg off the floor and extend it so it's straight, and then tap your heel on the floor.

    d.   Return your foot to the starting position, and then repeat for the other leg.

4. TVA leg lifts

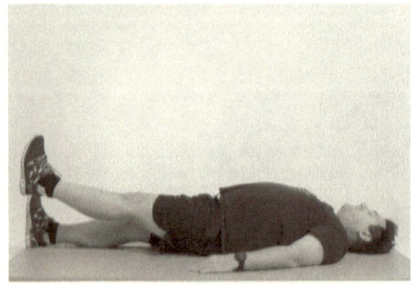 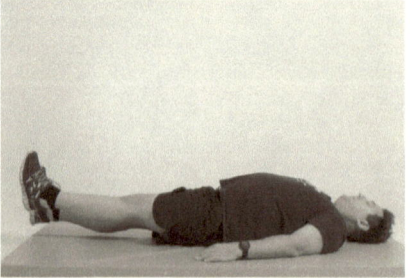

    a.   Lie on the floor on your back with your knees bent.

b. Turn on your pelvic floor by drawing it up as if preventing yourself from going to the bathroom. (Keep the pelvic floor turned on the whole time.)

c. Slowly lift one foot 2–3 cm. off the floor. As you put it back on the floor, lift the other foot off the floor (just before the first one touches the floor).

d. Make sure you don't arch your back as you change feet. If you need to do so, alternate feet if you're feeling pain.

5. Lower abdominals

a. Lie on your back with your knees bent and your feet close to your hips.

b. Place your hand in the curve of your lower back.

c. Flatten out your back so you're pressing your spine down on your hand.

d. Keeping the pressure on your hand, lift one foot off the floor, put it back on the floor, and then alternate sides.

e. Try to keep the same pressure on your hand the whole time. (You'll feel this in your lower abdominals.)

6. Wall stance

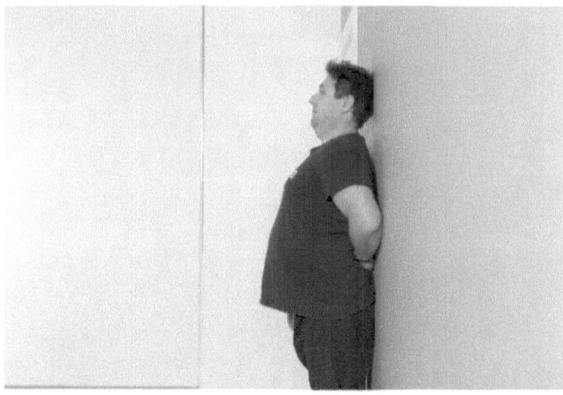

a. Stand with your heel, hips, shoulders, and head against the wall as shown above. Your posture may not allow you to do this. If so, focus on either the lower or upper part of the spine.

b. Place your hand behind your back until your knuckles are under your vertebrae.

c. Imagine you have headlights on your backside. Turn them down towards your heels. This will reduce the excessive curve in the spine. Hold your pelvis in this position for 30–45 seconds. Repeat 4–5 times throughout the day.

STRETCHES TO ASSIST WITH FLAT BACK

1. Hamstrings

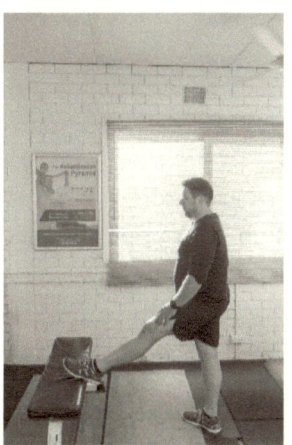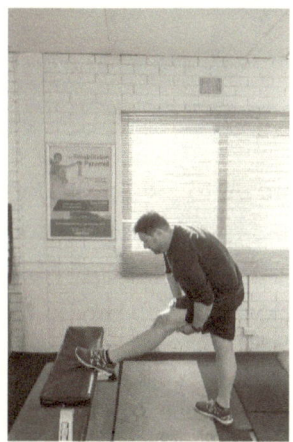

a. Place your foot on a step/bench.
b. Keep your knee slightly bent.
c. Bow forwards, tilting your hips up towards the ceiling. You should feel a stretch in the hamstring.

2. Glutes

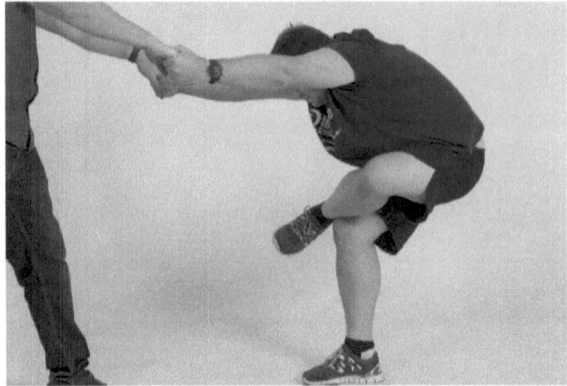

a. Hold on to a solid support for balance.
b. Cross your leg so your foot is on your opposite knee.
c. Leaning back, bend your knee as you allow yourself to sink backwards. You should feel the stretch in your backside.

3. Calf

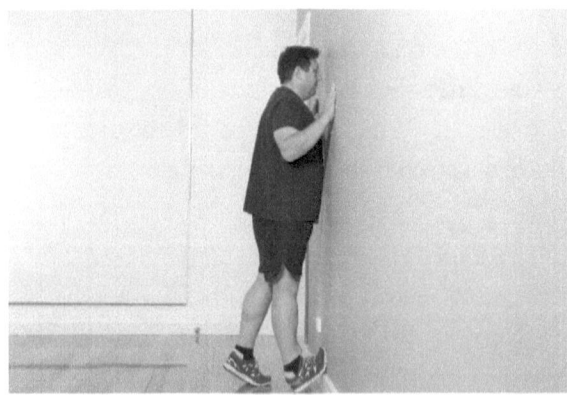

a. Stand tall. Place your foot against a wall or solid surface, with toes aimed at the ceiling.
b. Push your hips into the wall/surface.
c. Try not to let your heel slip backwards. You should feel a stretch in the calf.

4. Hip flexor

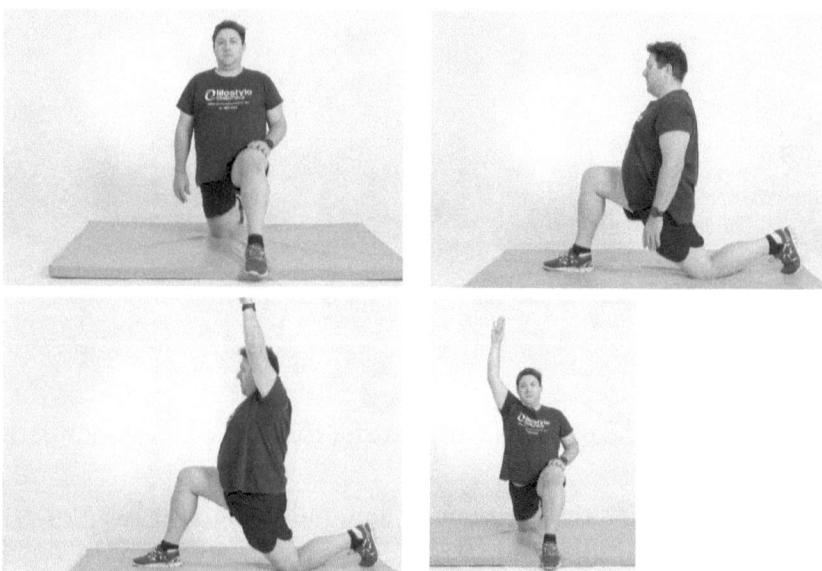

a. Kneel on the floor with one foot forward. (Make sure the foot is in front of the knee.)

b. Rock your weight forwards while keeping your hips tucked under your body.

c. Once your weight is over the front leg, lift the arm over your head (the opposite arm to the one that is forward).

5. Quads

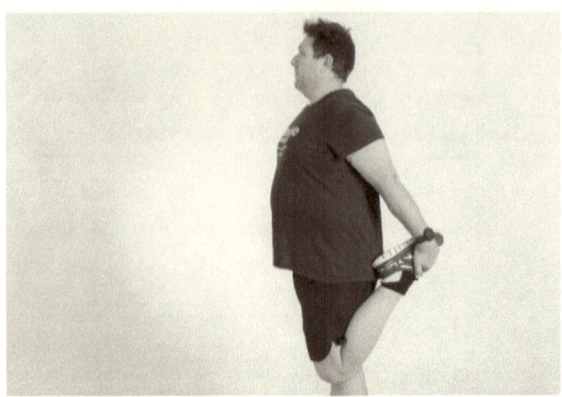

a. Holding on to a stable structure for balance, lift one leg towards your backside.
b. Holding on to your ankle or foot, pull up to your backside.
c. Keep your knees together and push your hips forwards. You'll feel the stretch in the front of the leg.

FORWARD HEAD CARRIAGE

WE CAN'T DISCUSS preventing and eliminating pain without looking to correct forward head carriage. By doing this program, you'll prevent headaches and neck stiffness and improve the range of movement in your neck.

Mobilisation and activation exercises that can help reduce excessive kyphosis are as follows:

1. Horizontal foam roller

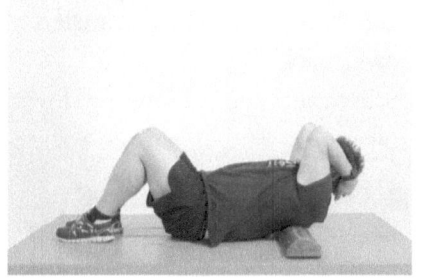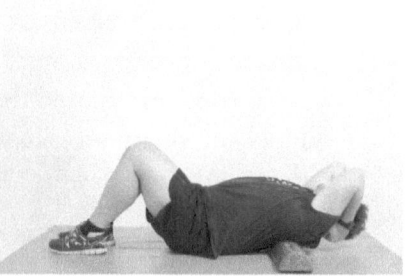

    a. Lie on your back with your knees bent. Place the D-shaped foam roller across your back at the height of the bottom of the shoulder blade (scapula).

    b. Place your hands behind your head, with your elbows pointing up towards the ceiling.

    c. As you breathe out, relax backwards (arching your back), only moving as far back as you can without any pain.

    d. As you breathe in, draw yourself up.

    e. Repeat three or four times, and then rest so the roller moves up your spine towards your head. As you move up the spine, it's like moving up only one segment of the vertebra at a time.

    f. Repeat the movements in steps c and d at each level of the vertebrae.

2. McKenzie press

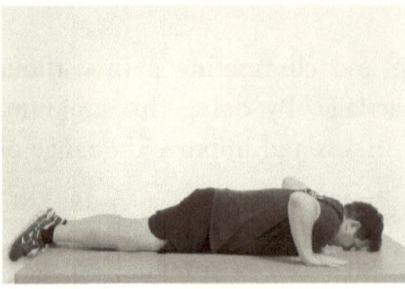 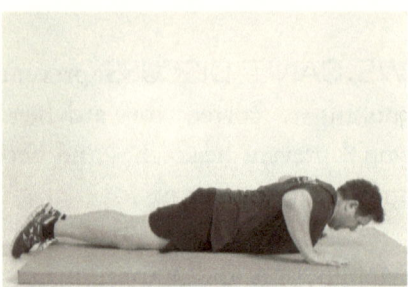

a. Lie on your stomach with your hands in the push-up position.

b. Push up through your arms so you take the weight out of your chest. (Note: you're not lifting from your lower back.)

c. Pull your shoulder blades back and together. Holding yourself up, take your weight out of your hands. Weight is transferred into the upper back, not the lower back.

d. Keep your chin tucked the whole time so you're looking down.

e. Hold for thirty seconds to start with, and repeat 2–4 times throughout the day.

3. Lewitt technique

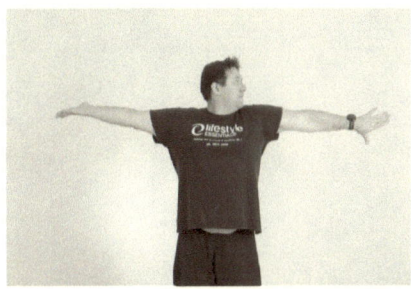 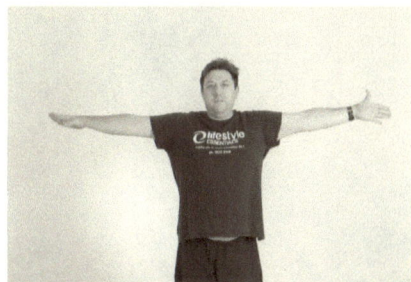

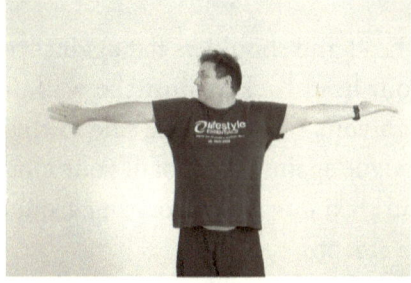

a. Stand or sit tall, with your arms straight to the side.
b. Point down the thumb of one arm to the floor while pointing up the other arm's palm towards the ceiling.
c. Look at the hand with the thumb pointing down.
d. Inhale deeply. As you breathe out, rotate your head from one side to the other, and simultaneously rotate your hands into the opposite position (thumb down turns to palm up, and the other moves from palm up to thumb down).
e. Breathe in and then rotate your head from side to side, simultaneously rotating your hands into the opposite position.

4. Chin tuck wall stance

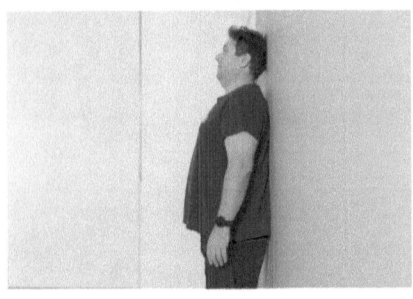 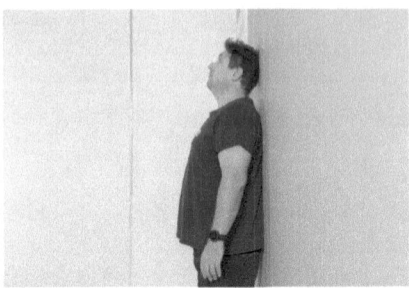

a. Lean your head and shoulders flat against the wall.
b. Holding your head back against the wall, imagine you have a pole through your ears from one side to the other.
c. Lift your tongue against the roof of your mouth; slowly roll your head up and then down as if rotating around the pole. (This is a small movement.)
d. Keep your head and shoulders against the wall the whole time.

Strength training programs need to be conducted in a neutral spine position. This means the head should remain in a chin-tuck position in all exercises (not looking up or forwards while lying down).

STRETCHES FOR FORWARD HEAD CARRIAGE

1. Pectoralis major stretch with mobilisation

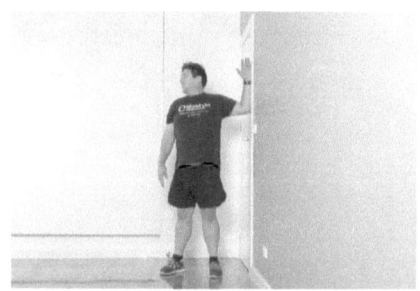 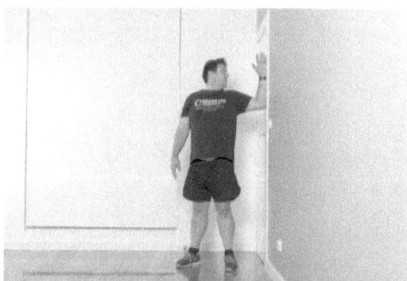

   a. Place your arm in a bent position, as shown in the diagram, against a wall, pole, or doorway.

   b. Keep the elbow at the same height as the shoulder.

   c. Rotate your body away from your arm so you feel the stretch through the chest.

   d. Looking at your hand, draw a deep breath.

   e. As you rotate your head to look away from your arm, breathe out.

2. Pectoralis minor chest stretch

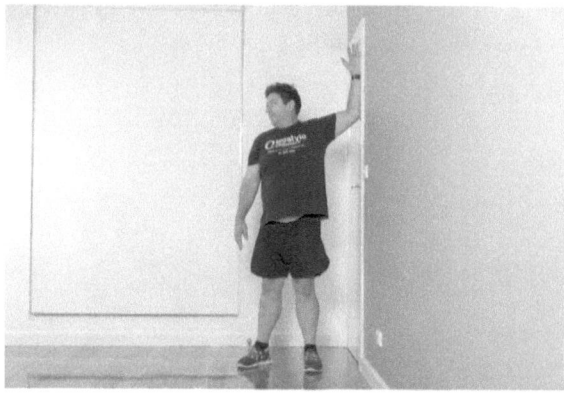

a. Place your arm in a bent position, as shown in the diagram, against a wall, pole, or doorway.
b. Place the elbow above the height of the shoulder.
c. Rotate your body away from your arm so you feel the stretch through the chest.
d. Looking at your hand, draw a deep breath.
e. As you rotate your head to look away from your arm, breathe out.

3. Lats (upper back) stretch

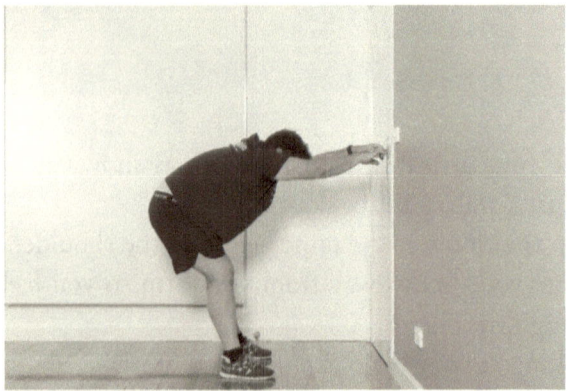

a. Hold on to a stable, solid object that can't move.
b. Sit back, taking the weight through your arms, bending your knees and bowing forwards, looking down towards the floor.
c. Holding on to the object, adjust your weight to one side of the body to stretch that side.
d. Change sides.

4. Upper trapezius stretch

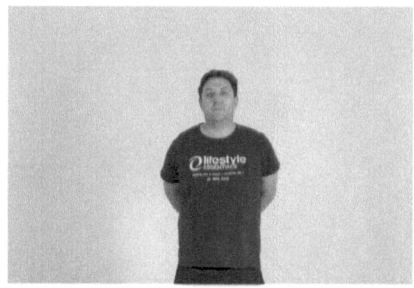
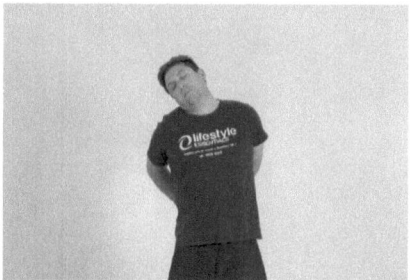
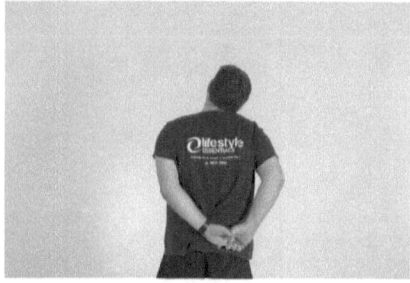

a. Sit on a chair nice and straight.
b. Hold on to the seat of the chair with one arm.
c. With the other arm, gently pull (tilt) your head in the opposite direction.
d. Once your head is tilted, you can rotate your head to find the most effective position to stretch the neck.

5. Levator stretch

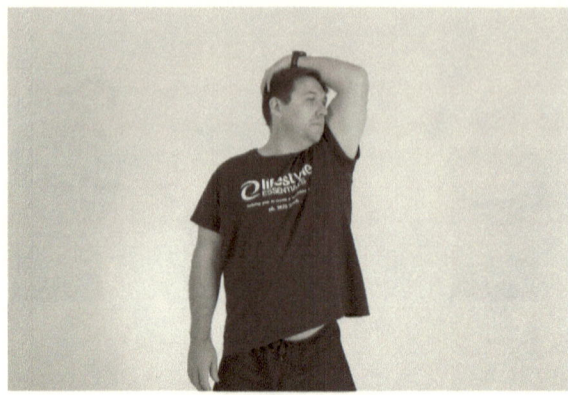

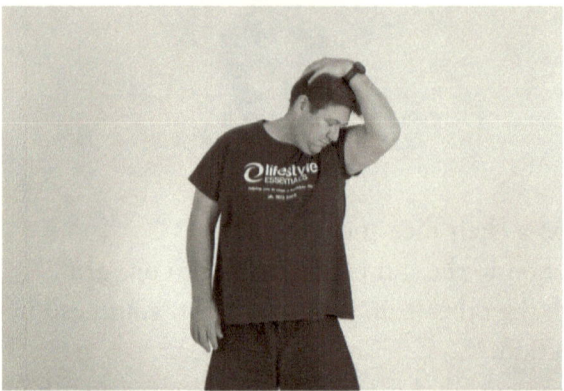

a. Sit or stand.
b. Turn your head as if you're looking down at your armpit.
c. Place your hand over your head as in the picture above.
d. Gently pull your head down to your armpit.
e. Turn on your core correctly.

When strengthening the core, it is has been suggested by Paul Chek that the abdominals respond to being trained in the following order:

1. TVA activation
2. rotation muscles
3. lower abdominals
4. full rectus abdominis (integration of all the abdominals)

SPECIFIC CORE STRENGTHENING EXERCISES

TVA

1. TVA heel taps

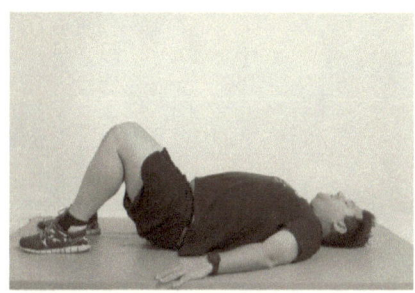 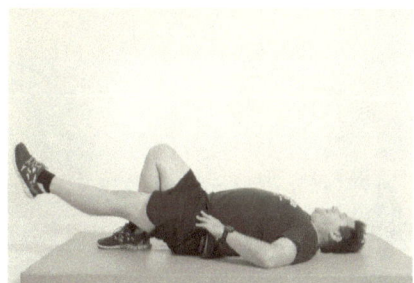

a. Lie on the floor on your back with your knee bent.
b. Turn on your pelvic floor by drawing it up as if preventing yourself from going to the bathroom. (Keep the pelvic floor turned on the whole time.)
c. Lift one leg off the floor and extend the leg out so it is straight, and then tap your heel on the floor.
d. Return your foot to the starting position; repeat on the other leg.

2. TVA hip flexion

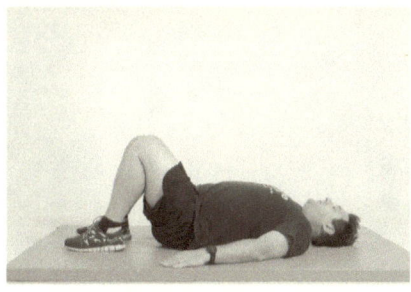 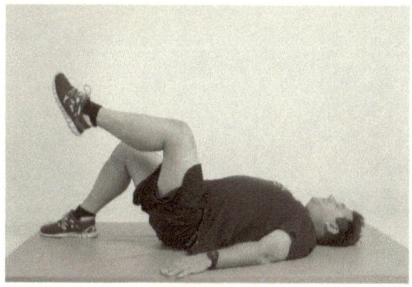

a. Lie on the floor on your back with your knee bent.

b. Turn on your pelvic floor by drawing it up as if preventing yourself from going to the bathroom. (Keep the pelvic floor turned on the whole time.)

c. Lift your foot off the floor from the hip.

d. Return it down, and lift the other one off the floor, alternating sides.

3. TVA leg lifts

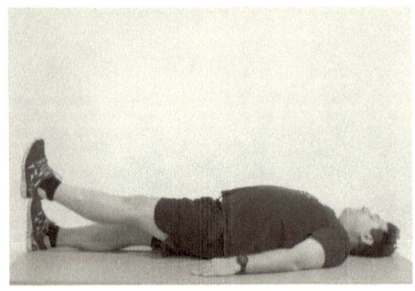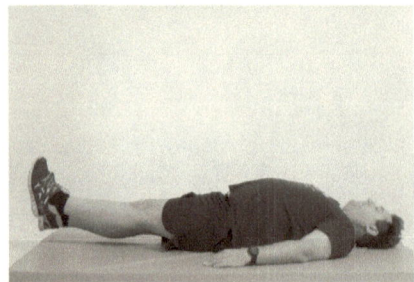

a. Lie on the floor on your back with your knees bent.

b. Turn on your pelvic floor by drawing it up as if preventing yourself from going to the bathroom. (Keep the pelvic floor turned on the whole time.)

c. Slowly lift one foot 2–3 cm. off the floor. As you put it back on the floor, lift the other foot off the floor (just before the first one touches the floor).

d. Make sure you don't arch your back as you change feet. If you need to do so, alternate feet if you're feeling pain.

Obliques

1. Russian twist (on back)

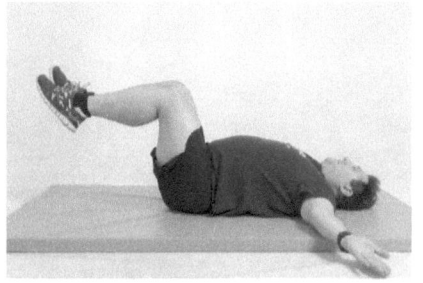
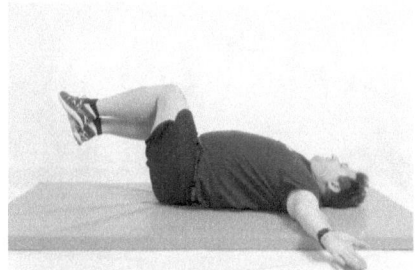
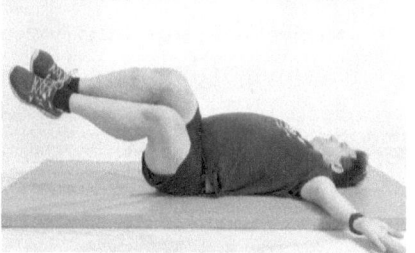

a. Lie on your back with your knees bent.
b. Keep your knees and feet together.
c. Rock the knees from one side to the other.
d. Let your feet lift off the ground as you rock from side to side.
e. Start with small movements that are slow and controlled.

2. Four-point stance (opposite extension)

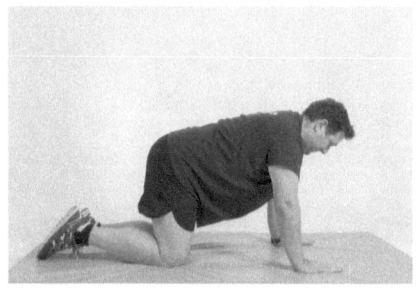
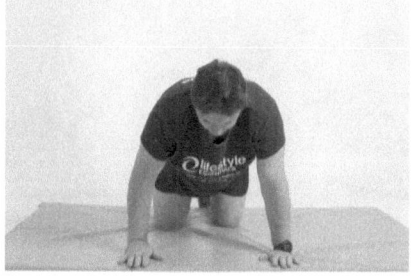

a. Activate your TVA by drawing in your abdomen.
b. Lift the opposite arm and leg, stretching them out straight. Try not to twist or arch your back.
c. Return to the floor, and then alternate sides.

3. Wood chops

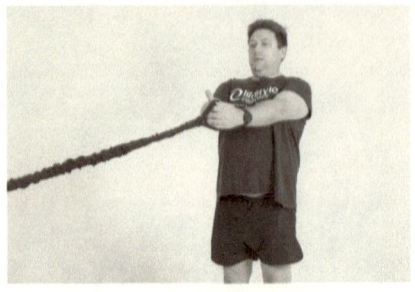 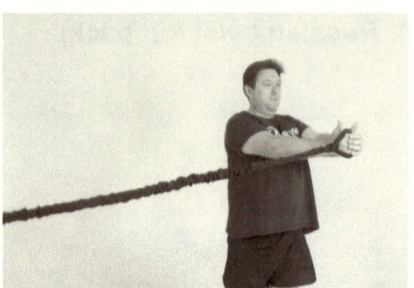

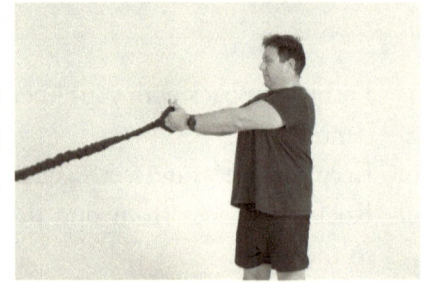

a. Stand up tall, holding on to a band or a cable.
b. Imagine your spine is a pole that can't bend in any direction. It remains upright the whole time.

4. Lower abdominals

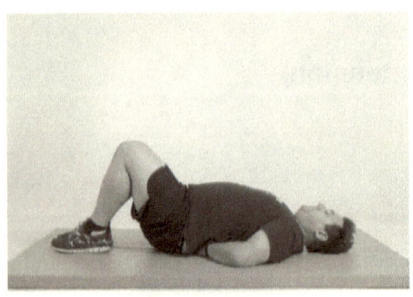 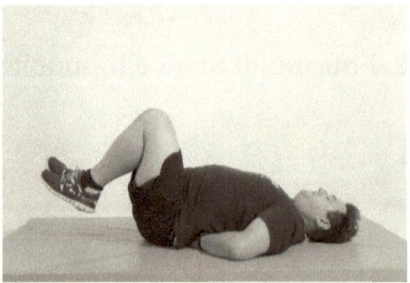

a. Lie on your back with your knees bent and your feet close to your hips.
b. Place your hand in the curve under your lower back.
c. Flatten out your back so you're pressing your spine down on your hand.
d. Keeping the pressure on your hand, lift one foot off the floor, return it to the floor, and alternate sides.

e. Try to keep the same pressure on your hand the whole time. (You'll feel this in your lower abdominals.)

Integrate with all abdominals

The plank

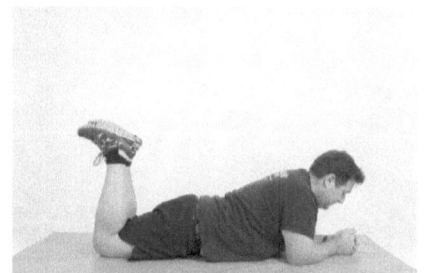
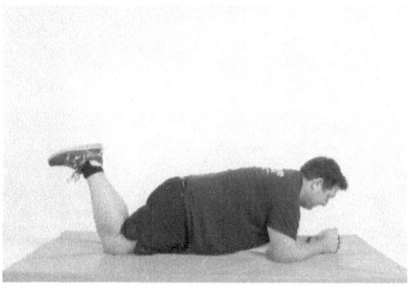
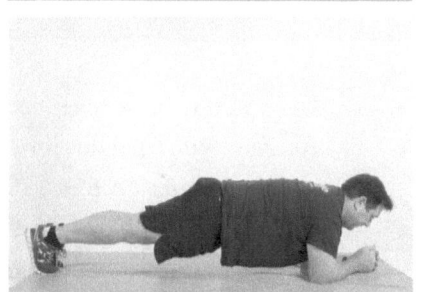

Step 4. Get your butt working

If your gluteal muscles don't work effectively, your lower back and hamstrings work harder to support the glutes. Over time, this leads to dysfunction either in the lower back or in the hamstrings. Furthermore, it can cause knee pain through patellar tracking issues. So getting your butt working properly is an essential part of any exercise program, whether you have back pain or you're an elite athlete who wishes to prevent injuries.

GLUTE ACTIVATION AND DEVELOPMENT SESSION

Gluteal activation

1. Hip extension holds

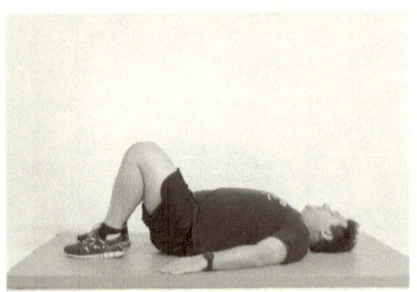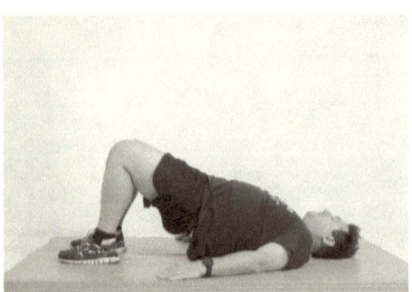

a.   Lie on your back with your knees bent.

b.   Activate your pelvic floor, and squeeze your butt muscles like you're holding on to a $100 bill.

c.   Once everything is activated, lift your hips off the floor. (Ideally, form a straight line from the shoulders to the knees. If you can't go this high, start at your own level.)

d.   Hold this position for thirty seconds. (Build up to thirty seconds if necessary.)

2. Hip extension thrusts

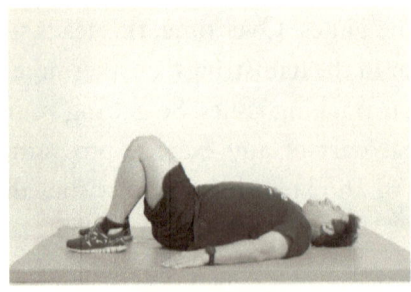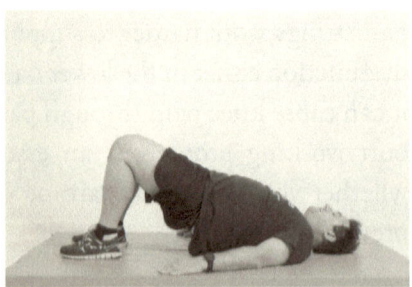

a.   Lie on your back with your knees bent, feet flat on the floor.

b. Activate your pelvic floor, and squeeze your butt muscles like you're holding on to a $100 bill.

c. Once everything is activated, lift your hips off the floor. (Ideally, form a straight line from the shoulders to the knees; but if you can't go this high, start at your own level.)

d. Return to the floor and relax, and then repeat from step b.

3. Posterior sling glute activation

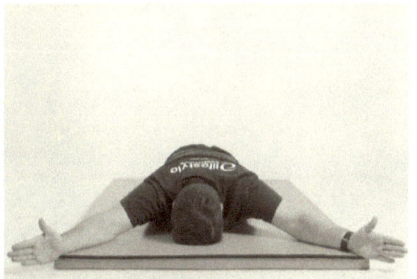 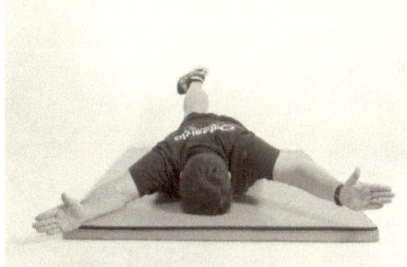

a. Lie on your stomach with your arms extended out on a forty-five-degree angle at the shoulder, pointing your thumbs up towards the ceiling.

b. Squeeze your glutes (butt), and lift your opposite arm and leg off the floor (2–3 cm) with your thumb pointing up.

c. Return to the floor.

d. Alternate sides.

SUMMARY

BACK PAIN IS an individual problem. A multitude of potential reasons and issues can cause back pain, some of which aren't even related to the back. The most important aspect of overcoming back pain is the *why*. Why do you have pain? If you don't have the *why*, then you'll never know what to do to eliminate or correct the problem. In saying this, after over twenty years of clinical experience, I know that the most important step in anyone's rehabilitation is to turn off the pain and then mobilise the neural system. These two steps alone will improve 90 per cent of people's issues. From this point, activating your glutes correctly and learning how to correctly activate the core will help strengthen and support the spine. This is essential in improving the quality of life and preventing all types of back pain and back conditions.

The final consideration with any musculoskeletal issue is to continue to move and strengthen the body once the pain has gone. This can be done by participating in a strength and conditioning program once or twice a week to prevent relapses and ensure that your functional levels don't become dysfunctional.

If you need more information or assistance with your rehabilitation or designing a proactive strength training program, contact us via our website, info@lifestyleessentials.com.au

More of these videos and exercises can be obtained through
www.stopbackpain.com.au/stop-back-pain-exercise-videos

www.ingramcontent.com/pod-product-compliance
Lightning Source LLC
Chambersburg PA
CBHW020519290526
45786CB00002B/670